Asthma: Nursing Care Across the Lifespan

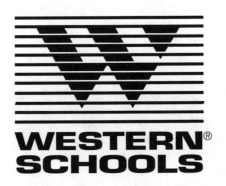

WESTERN® SCHOOLS

By
Anne Meng, MN, CPNP, RNC, AE-C

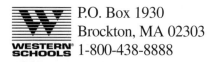

P.O. Box 1930
Brockton, MA 02303
1-800-438-8888

ABOUT THE AUTHOR

Anne Meng, MN, CPNP, RNC, AE-C, is an clinical nurse specialist and advanced nurse practitioner in the Department of Women's, Infant's and Children's Nursing and Special Projects Coordinator for the Children's Hospital at the University of Texas Medical Branch, Galveston Texas. Ms. Meng has extensive experience in the nursing care of children and their families. She practices as a pediatric nurse practitioner in a children's asthma clinic, founded and directs an educationally based children's asthma camp, and has been the principal investigator for camp-related outcome studies. The camp is a model camp and has been successfully replicated in another community.

Ms. Meng has extensive teaching experience in baccalaureate and masters nursing programs as well as in nursing staff development programs. She has designed innovative interactive nurse preceptor programs as part of a nursing initiative for staff development. She has numerous asthma related publications and is a founding member of the Asthma Coalition of Texas.

Dedication: This book is dedicated to my niece, Michelle, who understands living with asthma.

Anne Meng has disclosed that she is the recipient of small grants from GlaxoSmithKline, Monaghan Medical Corporation, AstraZeneca and the University of British Columbia Pharmacology & Therapeutics.

ABOUT THE SUBJECT MATTER REVIEWER

Christine Wagner, RN, MSN, CPNP, FNP-BC, AE-C, is board certified as a pediatric and family nurse practitioner and as an asthma educator. She has over 25 years of experience in the field of asthma and allergy. Ms. Wagner obtained her bachelor's and master's degrees in nursing from the University of Texas Health Science Center at Houston and completed a postmaster's program at Houston Baptist University.

Ms. Wagner has developed and presented numerous educational programs on asthma, allergic diseases, and patient education across the country, and she has published multiple articles about these topics. She is an active member of the American Academy and College of Allergy, Asthma, and Immunology, attending and conducting educational programs with both organizations. Ms. Wagner is a founding member and the first president of the Association of Asthma Educators and past vice-chair for the National Asthma Educator Certification Board.

Christine Wagner has disclosed that she has no significant financial or other conflicts of interest pertaining to this course book.

Nurse Planner: Amy Bernard, RN, BSN, MS

Copy Editor: Liz Schaeffer

Indexer: Sylvia Coates

ISBN: 1-57801-135-3

IMPORTANT: Read these instructions *BEFORE* proceeding!

Enclosed with your course book, you will find the FasTrax® answer sheet. Use this form to answer all the final exam questions that appear in this course book. If you are completing more than one course, be sure to write your answers on the appropriate answer sheet. Full instructions and complete grading details are printed on the FasTrax instruction sheet, also enclosed with your order. Please review them before starting. *If you are mailing your answer sheet(s) to Western Schools, we recommend you make a copy as a backup.*

ABOUT THIS COURSE

A Pretest is provided with each course to test your current knowledge base regarding the subject matter contained within this course. Your Final Exam is a multiple choice examination. **You will find the exam questions at the end of each chapter.**

In the event the course has less than 100 questions, leave the remaining answer boxes on the FasTrax answer sheet blank. **Use a <u>black</u> pen to fill in your answer sheet.**

A PASSING SCORE

You must score 70% or better in order to pass this course and receive your Certificate of Completion. Should you fail to achieve the required score, we will send you an additional FasTrax answer sheet so that you may make a second attempt to pass the course. Western Schools will allow you three chances to pass the same course…*at no extra charge!* After three failed attempts to pass the same course, your file will be closed.

RECORDING YOUR HOURS

Please monitor the time it takes to complete this course using the handy log sheet on the other side of this page. See below for transferring study hours to the course evaluation.

COURSE EVALUATIONS

In this course book, you will find a short evaluation about the course you are soon to complete. This information is vital to providing Western Schools with feedback on this course. The course evaluation answer section is in the lower right hand corner of the FasTrax answer sheet marked "Evaluation," with answers marked 1–23. Your answers are important to us; please take a few minutes to complete the evaluation.

On the back of the FasTrax instruction sheet, there is additional space to make any comments about the course, the school, and suggested new curriculum. Please mail the FasTrax instruction sheet, with your comments, back to Western Schools in the envelope provided with your course order.

TRANSFERRING STUDY TIME

Upon completion of the course, transfer the total study time from your log sheet to question 23 in the course evaluation. The answers will be in ranges; please choose the proper hour range that best represents your study time. You **MUST** log your study time under question 23 on the course evaluation.

EXTENSIONS

You have two (2) years from the date of enrollment to complete this course. A six (6) month extension may be purchased. If after 30 months from the original enrollment date you do not complete the course, *your file will be closed and no certificate can be issued.*

CHANGE OF ADDRESS?

In the event you have moved during the completion of this course, please call our student services department at 1-800-618-1670, and we will update your file.

A GUARANTEE TO WHICH YOU'LL GIVE HIGH HONORS

If any continuing education course fails to meet your expectations or if you are not satisfied in any manner, for any reason, you may return it for an exchange or a refund (less shipping and handling) within 30 days. Software, video, and audio courses must be returned unopened.

Thank you for enrolling at Western Schools!

WESTERN SCHOOLS
P.O. Box 1930
Brockton, MA 02303
(800) 438-8888
www.westernschools.com

Asthma:
Nursing Care Across the Lifespan

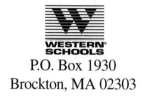

WESTERN SCHOOLS

P.O. Box 1930
Brockton, MA 02303

Please use this log to total the number of hours you spend reading the text and taking the final examination.

Date	Hours Spent
1/26 1/27	1 ~ 1
2/2	1
2/6	1
2/14	2 .5
	3
	1
	.5
	1
	1
	1

TOTAL | 20

Please log your study hours with submission of your final exam. To log your study time, fill in the appropriate circle under question 23 of the FasTrax® answer sheet under the "Evaluation" section.

Asthma:
Nursing Care Across the Lifespan

WESTERN SCHOOLS
CONTINUING EDUCATION EVALUATION

Instructions: Mark your answers to the following questions with a black pen on the "Evaluation" section of your FasTrax® answer sheet provided with this course. You should not return this sheet.

Please use the scale below to rate how well the course content met the educational objectives.

A	Agree Strongly	C	Disagree Somewhat
B	Agree Somewhat	D	Disagree Strongly

After completing this course I am able to

1. Recognize asthma as a major public health problem across all age-groups.

2. Recognize the impact of asthma as a chronic inflammatory disease on the role of the nurse when teaching patients the importance of anti-inflammatory medication for optimal asthma control.

3. Recognize the diagnostic approach to asthma and the nurse's role in case finding.

4. Recognize the role of symptom and peak flow monitoring in the management of asthma.

5. Identify the role of quick-relief and long-term controller medications in the management of asthma and provide patient and family education related to optimal use of asthma medications.

6. Recognize common asthma triggers and provide education regarding basic environmental control to patients and families.

7. Recognize how the child's stage of development impacts (or influences) asthma management.

8. Identify how the course of asthma changes during pregnancy and how these changes impact asthma management.

9. Recognize unique features of asthma in adults and how comorbid conditions and the aging process affect the care of older adults with asthma.

10. Recognize signs and symptoms of an acute asthma attack and apply appropriate nursing interventions.

11. Identify signs and symptoms of exercise-induced asthma (EIA) and provide basic education to the patient and family regarding control of EIA and participation in sports.

12. Recognize the impact of comorbid diseases such as atopic dermatitis, allergic rhinitis, sinusitis, and gastroesophageal reflux on optimal asthma control.

13. Recognize asthma education as a critical component of comprehensive asthma management and identify appropriate asthma teaching content and strategies in various clinical contexts.

14. Recognize the role of written self-management plans in the overall plan of care and identify design characteristics that enhance the usefulness of these tools.

15. Recognize the unique benefits of asthma education in the camp setting for children with asthma and their parents.

16. Identify the nurse's role in educating patients with asthma and their families about alternative therapies and their impact on asthma.

17. The content of this course was relevant to the objectives.

18. This offering met my professional education needs.

19. The objectives met the overall purpose/goal of the course.

20. The course was generally well-written and the subject matter explained thoroughly. (If no, please explain on the back of the FasTrax instruction sheet.)

21. The content of this course was appropriate for home study.

22. The final examination was well-written and at an appropriate level for the content of the course.

23. **PLEASE LOG YOUR STUDY HOURS WITH SUBMISSION OF YOUR FINAL EXAM.**
   Please choose which best represents the total study hours it took to complete this 28-hour course.

   A. Less than 23 hours   C. 27–30 hours
   B. 23–26 hours   D. Greater than 30 hours

CONTENTS

FIGURES AND TABLES

PRETEST

1. Begin this course by taking the pretest. Circle the answers to the questions on this page, or write the answers on a separate sheet of paper. Do not log answers to the pretest questions on the FasTrax test sheet included with the course.

2. Compare your answers to the PRETEST KEY located in the back of the book. The pretest answer key indicates the course chapter where the content of that question is discussed. Make note of the questions you missed, so that you can focus on those areas as you complete the course.

3. Complete the course by reading each chapter and completing the exam questions at the end of the chapter. Answers to these exam questions should be logged on the FasTrax test sheet included with the course.

1. In recent years, prevalence rates of asthma have increased in

    a. developed countries.

    b. underdeveloped countries.

    c. rural areas.

    d. mountainous regions.

2. The disease classification of asthma is

    a. acute.

    b. recurrent.

    c. chronic.

    d. infectious.

3. Diagnosis of asthma is related to

    a. severity of symptoms.

    b. age of the patient.

    c. level of eosinophils in the blood.

    d. duration of symptoms.

4. Peak flow meters are useful as

    a. a diagnostic tool.

    b. a motivating strategy for patients.

    c. an indicator of inspiratory effort.

    d. a monitoring tool.

5. Optimal control of asthma is achieved with the class of medications known as

    a. inhaled corticosteroids.

    b. bronchodilators.

    c. anticholinergics.

    d. leukotrienes.

6. A patient has recently begun using albuterol every day. This is an indication that

    a. the patient understands principles of medication adjustment.

    b. the patient's asthma is out of control.

    c. the patient needs to be hospitalized.

    d. the patient needs to avoid triggers.

7. The most common trigger for patients with asthma is

    a. mold.

    b. dust.

    c. cat dander.

    d. smoke.

8. The best trigger control strategy for smoke is to

    a. smoke outside of the house.

    b. smoke in a confined area of the house.

    c. stop smoking.

    d. ventilate the house when smoking.

9. Children tend to outgrow asthma

    a. by age 6.

    b. by age 12.

    c. by age 18.

    d. never.

10. The most severe asthma episodes in children are usually triggered by

    a. smoke.

    b. viral infections.

    c. bacterial infections.

    d. mold.

11. A woman with asthma tells the nurse she is pregnant. The nurse should advise the patient to

    a. stop using controller medication.

    b. decrease her controller medication by half.

    c. avoid allergy medication.

    d. continue taking her controller medication.

12. An adult with asthma experiences runny nose and congestion after taking aspirin. The nurse should interpret this as

    a. a sign of concurrent upper respiratory infection.

    b. unrelated to asthma.

    c. a sign of aspirin sensitivity.

    d. an insignificant event.

13. An older adult with asthma is hypertensive. The nurse should advise the patient to avoid

    a. beta-agonists.

    b. ACE inhibitors.

    c. thiazide diuretics.

    d. beta-blockers.

14. A person with asthma is seen in the emergency department an average of three times per year with moderately severe attacks. The nurse should interpret this as an indication

    a. for hospitalization.

    b. that asthma is out of control.

    c. that severe attacks cannot be avoided.

    d. for referral to a specialist.

15. The school nurse receives a note from a parent requesting that her child with asthma be excused from physical education. The best response of the nurse is to

    a. honor the request.

    b. ask the mother to have the child evaluated by a specialist.

    c. reinforce the request by teaching the child to participate in quiet activities.

    d. explain the importance of physical fitness to the mother.

16. The nurse sees a patient with uncontrolled asthma and chronic runny nose. The nurse should recognize that the patient's runny nose is

    a. part of the same inflammatory process that occurs in the lower airway.

    b. uncomfortable but unrelated to asthma.

    c. limiting the patient's ability to use inhaled medications.

    d. a side effect of asthma medications.

17. The best strategy for providing education to the person with asthma is to

    a. refer the patient to group classes.

    b. provide teaching in steps at each visit.

    c. include all teaching in one extended clinic visit.

    d. refer the patient to Internet sources.

18. According to the National Asthma Education and Prevention Program, written self-management plans are a component of care for

    a. all patients.

    b. patients with asthma that is difficult to control.

    c. pediatric patients.

    d. patients with moderate to severe persistent asthma.

19. Children most likely to benefit from an asthma camp program include those

    a. between ages 5 and 6.

    b. with learning impairments.

    c. with mild intermittent asthma.

    d. who miss school frequently because of asthma.

20. The percent of patients with asthma who use alternative therapies is approximately

    a. 5%.

    b. 15%.

    c. 27%.

    d. 40%.

INTRODUCTION

Rates of asthma have increased dramatically since the early 1980s. The National Centers for Disease Control and Prevention (CDC) estimates that between 1980 and 1996, the incidence of asthma increased 73.9%, affecting 14.6 million persons in the United States. Asthma occurs in all ages and ethnic groups, but its incidence is highest among children ages 5 to 14 years, African Americans, and women (CDC, 2002). The CDC further reports that asthma-related work and school absences have increased 50% and now account for 14 million lost work and school days. Because of this dramatic increase, asthma is now recognized as a national public health problem.

Our understanding of the nature of asthma as an inflammatory airway disease has increased greatly in recent years. Accompanying this understanding are improvements in diagnostic guidelines and medications. Studies of indoor and outdoor pollutants have added to our knowledge of asthma triggers. Evidenced-based guidelines for managing asthma are now available to assist the healthcare provider in delivering optimal asthma care (National Heart, Lung, and Blood Institute, 1997).

Because asthma is a chronic disease that occurs across all age-groups, nurses in virtually every setting can expect to care for clients with asthma. Increasingly, asthma is seen in adults, in the elderly, in school-age children, in occupational settings, and in the pregnant woman. Recent advances in our understanding of asthma and its treatment have implications for continuing education of all nurses. Other healthcare professionals can also benefit from this course.

The purpose of this course is to provide an overview of asthma; discuss differences in how asthma affects children, the pregnant woman, adults, and the elderly; and describe related nursing care. The pathology of asthma, disease symptoms, environmental triggers, diagnosis, treatment, associated conditions, and health education are discussed.

REFERENCES

Centers for Disease Control and Prevention. (2002). Surveillance for asthma — United States, 1980-1999. *Morbidity and Mortality Weekly Report. 51*(SS01), 1-13.

National Heart, Lung, and Blood Institute; National Asthma Education and Prevention Program. Expert panel report 2. (1997). *Guidelines for the diagnosis and management of asthma.* (NIH Pub No. 97-4051). Bethesda, MD: National Institute of Health; National Heart, Lung, and Blood Institite. Available online at http://www.nhlbi.nih.gov/guidelines/asthma/asthgdln.pdf

CHAPTER 1

EPIDEMIOLOGY OF ASTHMA

CHAPTER OBJECTIVE

Upon completion of this chapter, the reader will be able to recognize asthma as a major public health problem across all age-groups.

LEARNING OBJECTIVES

After studying this chapter, the reader will be able to

1. recognize the trend of increasing asthma prevalence.

2. identify two groups at high risk for asthma mortality.

3. identify two groups at high risk for developing asthma.

4. recognize the cost burden of asthma.

5. relate high prevalence of asthma to environmental concerns.

6. identify five national goals for the management of asthma.

HISTORICAL TRENDS IN ASTHMA PREVALENCE

Prevalence rates of asthma have increased dramatically since the early 1980s, prompting some to label this trend as an "epidemic" (Petronella, & Conboy-Ellis, 2003). Data on asthma rates are collected by self-report through the Centers for Disease Control and Prevention National Health Interview Survey. As self-reported material, prevalence data are estimates. Strategies for improving surveillance are being developed (Centers for Disease Control and Prevention [CDC], 2002a).

Between 1980 and 1996 rates of asthma cases increased 73.9%, representing an estimated 14.6 million persons reporting asthma during the previous year. In 2001, an astounding 31.3 million people reported a physician diagnosis of asthma in their lifetime (National Center for Health Statistics [NCHS], 2004). Between 1980 and 1996, the number of school and work absences increased slightly more than 50%, representing a total of 14 million occurrences each. This increase is consistent with the increased prevalence of asthma because missed school and workdays per individuals known to have asthma remained stable (CDC, 2002a). Between 1980 and 1999, the number of persons visiting a healthcare provider for a primary diagnosis of asthma increased from 5.9 million to 10.8 million (CDC, 2004). Nationally, hospitalization rates for asthma peaked in the mid-1980s and gradually declined since then; however, regional differences exist. For example, hospitalization rates have increased in the Northeast, whereas they declined in the Western United States (CDC, 2004). Emergency room (ER) visits increased by a rate of 29% between 1992 and 1999, with highest rates recorded in the northeastern United States (CDC, 2004).

Internationally, asthma is on the increase, but incidence varies among different populations. The greatest increases have been reported in Australia, New Zealand, and England. It is not yet clear whether the differences in asthma rates are due to industrialization, environment, or exposure to different allergen loads, but higher asthma rates are reported in developed countries, leading some to suspect that lifestyle is a factor contributing to the increase (National Heart, Lung, and Blood Institute, World Health Organization [NHLBI/WHO], 2003).

Asthma, as an "epidemic" is a major public health problem and is a key component of the Healthy People 2010 objectives (U.S. Department of Health and Human Services, [DHHS], 2000). National goals for managing asthma include reducing asthma (a) deaths, (b) hospitalizations, (c) emergency room visits, (d) activity limitations, (e) and missed work or school days. Management goals also include increasing the number of persons with asthma who receive formal patient education and healthcare that is consistent with the National Asthma Education and Prevention Program's (NAEPP, 1997) guidelines and referral to community and self-help resources. The NAEPP guidelines represent a consensus of asthma experts and are the foundation to the development of this continuing education program. The NAEPP guidelines will be reviewed in greater detail throughout this module.

ASTHMA MORTALITY

Death rates for asthma increased gradually during the period from 1980 to 1995, but they appear to be leveling or even declining. Data for 1998 indicate a mortality rate of 2.0 per 100,000 persons, or 5,438 Americans. This rate declined in 1999. Death rates vary by region of the country and are highest in the western region of the United States. These rates also vary by group and are high among African Americans, women, and especially high among the elderly (CDC, 2002a).

It has been suggested that the asthma-related mortality in the United States is underestimated. This increase is puzzling but may be explained by an overall increase in the severity of asthma, failure to manage asthma—particularly failure to use anti-inflammatory medication, and overuse of short-acting beta$_2$-agonists (NHLBI/WHO, 2003).

RISK FACTORS FOR THE DEVELOPMENT OF ASTHMA

Age

Children

Children are at high risk for developing asthma. In 1996, the estimated prevalence of asthma in children younger than age 14 was 3,576,000. In 1996, 3,113,000 children younger than age 14 reported an attack in the last year. History of asthma attack in the past year is used as a marker of uncontrolled asthma. This means that more than 3 million children are at high risk for hospitalization or ER visits (CDC, 2002b). In children, asthma rates are 30% higher in boys than in girls (NCHS, 2004).

Currently, asthma is the leading chronic illness of childhood and the major cause of missed school days, accounting for 14 million absences annually. The greatest increase in asthma rates is seen in children ages 5 to 14 years, but asthma has also increased greatly in children younger than age 5. These youngest children have the highest ER and hospitalization rates (NCHS, 2004).

Young children are particularly at risk for developing asthma if their parents smoke (NHLBI/WHO, 2003). Second hand smoke is more toxic than directly inhaled smoke. Smoking during pregnancy and any smoking in the household after the child is born increases childhood risk of asthma.

Adults

At one time asthma was considered a childhood disease but this is no longer true. As shown in Table 1-1, asthma is increasing across all age-groups. Much of the increase in adults is attributed to an increase in occupational or work-related asthma and the development of allergy. Among adults, asthma affects more women than men. Rates are especially high among the elderly. Data from the Nurses Health Study suggest a higher incidence of asthma in postmenopausal women taking estrogen (NHLBI/WHO, 2003).

Ethnicity

African Americans are at highest risk for asthma and uncontrolled asthma. Rates of asthma for African Americans in 2001 exceeded rates for whites by 10% and exceeded rates for Hispanics by 40% (NCHS, 2004). The number of ER visits for African Americans in 2000 was 125% higher than for whites, hospitalization rates were 220% higher than in whites, and death rates were 200% higher than in whites (NCHS, 2004).

Interestingly, in a recent survey of ethnicity (CDC, 2004), highest asthma rates were not reported among African Americans. Rates were highest among non-Hispanics of multiple races (15.6%), followed by Native Americans (11.6%), African Americans (9.3%), Whites (7.6%), and Hispanics (5.0%). Puerto Ricans reported higher rates (11.6%) than other Hispanic respondents. These data indicate that markers of uncontrolled asthma such as ER visits do not mirror prevalence rates by ethnicity. In addition to extremely high ER visits in African Americans, ER visits for Hispanics and non-Hispanic multiracial respondents are disproportionately high when compared with ER visits for whites. These groups also

TABLE 1-1: ESTIMATED ANNUAL NUMBER OF PERSONS WITH ASTHMA IN THE PRECEDING 12 MONTHS, FROM 1980-1999

	1980 Self-Report of Asthma*	1999 Self-Report of Asthma in last 12 months
Race		
White	5,975,000	8,226,000
African American	899,000	1,535,000
Other 102,000	727,000	
Sex		
Male	3,438,000	4,310,000
Female	3,538,000	6,178,000
Age-groups		
0-4 years	369,000	825,000
5-14 years	1,530,000	2,288,000
15-34 years	2,251,000	3,208.000
35-64 years	2,056,000	3,451.000
> 65 years	769,000	717,000
Total	6,975,000	10,488,000

* National Health Interview Survey data - interview question changed slightly between 1980 and 1999.

Note. From Centers for Disease Control and Prevention. Surveillance for Asthma—United States, 1980-1999. *Morbidity and Mortality Weekly Report.* *51*(5501), 1-13.

reported increased negative indicators of control, such as more frequent urgent care visits, increased symptoms, nocturnal asthma, and activity limitations. Whites and Asians were the least likely to visit the ER and exhibited the most positive asthma control profiles. These indicators reflect healthcare disparities. These data are important to consider when developing or evaluating asthma programs and interventions.

COST OF ASTHMA

The cost of medical treatments for asthma can represent a substantial proportion of family income and federal expenditure. The estimated costs to families range from 5.5% to 14.5% of total family income (NHLBI/WHO, 2003). In 1998, asthma care cost the United States an estimated $12.7 billion (Weiss, & Sullivan, 2001). The most expensive form of care is acute care in the ER or hospital. The average cost of an ER visit is $248 for children younger than age 5, and $457 for adults. Average hospital costs are $3,103, but can be as high as $15,000. Overuse of short acting beta$_2$-agonists is predictive of high asthma costs. Cost for asthma care was found to be 24% higher for African American children than for white children. These data reflect frequent ER and hospital visits among African American children (Weiss & Sullivan, 2001).

It is well established that primary care is more cost effective than hospitalization and ER care. Primary care interventions have been shown to improve the diagnosis and treatment of children with asthma and reduce cost of care (Meng, 2000; Griffiths et al., 2004). Primary care by an educated nurse is associated with favorable outcomes but the intensity of the interventions needs to be sustained over time. Nurses at every point in the healthcare system have a role in supporting asthma management goals by providing and continually reinforcing patient and family education.

ENVIRONMENTAL CONCERNS

There have been hundreds of reports on the increasing prevalence of asthma in developed countries around the world. Asthma rates are especially high in urban areas. A concept, termed the "Hygiene Hypothesis" has been developed to explain the differences in asthma prevalence between rural and urbanized areas. This hypothesis holds that a sanitized lifestyle and reliance on antibiotics leads to an imbalance in the immune system, favoring the development of asthma. There is evidence that persons living on farms and religious groups who avoid antibiotics and immunizations suffer less asthma. However, more data are needed to confirm this hypothesis (NHLBI/WHO, 2003).

It is well known that asthma has a genetic component, but the dramatic increase in prevalence in such a short timespan points to environment to explain this increase. Recently, there has been an increase in research spending to examine the effect of indoor environmental triggers on asthma. This is reasonable because most people with asthma spend considerable time indoors, and indoor environments are easier to control than outdoor environments (Institute of Medicine, 2000).

Outdoor pollution is difficult to study and control; however, new strategies for measuring of outdoor pollution are leading to better scientific methodologies. Research in this area is increasing also. Recent data from these studies indicate that pollution is indeed a factor contributing to the severity of the asthma problem (NHLBI/WHO, 2003). To help the patient and family successfully manage asthma, the nurse must include education regarding environmental control in the plan of care.

SUMMARY

Dramatic increases in prevalence rates have led to labeling asthma as an epidemic, or major national health problem. The epidemiology of asthma has been the focus of numerous governmental reports. The modern lifestyle is associated with increased indoor and outdoor triggers and is thought to explain the increased asthma prevalence. National goals for managing asthma have been identified, but health programs must address disparities in care as evidenced by high healthcare utilization and death rates for minority groups.

High rates of asthma present a significant cost burden to families and the nation. Care needs to shift from costly ER visits and hospitalizations to primary care sites. Educated nurses can positively affect asthma care outcomes in every healthcare setting.

EXAM QUESTIONS

CHAPTER 1
Questions 1-6

1. National goals for managing asthma include

    a. referral of all persons with asthma to a specialist.

    b. monthly primary care visits.

    c. reduced ER visits and hospitalizations.

    d. administration of the influenza vaccine as a preventive measure.

2. Healthy People 2010 recommends that health-care for persons with asthma should be consistent with the guidelines known as the

    a. Center for Disease Control Asthma Plan.

    b. National Asthma Education and Prevention Program.

    c. Global Initiative for Asthma.

    d. Institute of Medicine's Environmental Control Plan.

3. A factor that has contributed to the increase of asthma in children under age 5 years is

    a. living on a farm.

    b. failure to use antibiotics.

    c. increased genetic mutation.

    d. parental smoking.

4. In planning asthma education programs, the nurse should be aware that the group at highest risk for poor asthma control is

    a. African Americans.

    b. Native Americans.

    c. Puerto Ricans.

    d. all of the above.

5. The recent increase in asthma prevalence can best be explained by

    a. improved diagnosis.

    b. environmental factors.

    c. increase in genetic mutations.

    d. the hygiene hypothesis.

6. The average estimated percent of income spent on asthma care by the family of a person with asthma is

    a. 1%.

    b. 10%.

    c. 20%.

    d. 40%.

7

REFERENCES

Centers for Disease Control and Prevention. (2002a). Surveillance for asthma — United States, 1980-1999. *Morbidity and Mortality Weekly Report. 51*(SS01), 1-13.

Centers for Disease Control and Prevention. (2002b). *New Asthma Estimates: Tracking prevalence, health care and mortality.* Retrieved July 18, 2004, from http://www.cdc.gov

Centers for Disease Control and Prevention. (2004). Asthma prevalence and control characteristics by race/ethnicity – United States, 2002. *Morbidity and Mortality Weekly Report, 53*(07), 145-148.

Griffiths, C., Foster, G., Barnes, N., Eldridge, S., Tate, H., Begum, S., et al. (2004). Specialist nurse intervention to reduce unscheduled asthma care in a deprived multiethnic area: The east London randomized controlled trial for high risk asthma (ELECTRA). *British Medical Journal* 2004, January 17; 328(7432): 144. doi: 10.1136/bjm.37950.784444.EE.

Institute of Medicine, Committee on the Assessment of Asthma and Indoor Air. (2000). *Clearing the air: Asthma and indoor exposures.* National Academy Press. Washington, D.C.

Meng, A. (2000). A school-based asthma clinic: A partnership model for managing childhood asthma. *Nurse Practitioner Forum, 11,* 38-47.

National Center for Health Statistics. (2004). *Asthma prevalence, health care use and mortality, 2000-2001.* Retrieved August 8, 2004 from http://www.cdc.gov/nchs/products/pubs/pubd/hestats/asthma

National Heart, Lung and Blood Institute/World Health Organization. (2003). *Global Initiative for Asthma: Global strategies for asthma management and prevention.* (NIH Publication No. 02-3659). Retrieved September 12, 2002, from http://www.ginasthma.com

National Asthma Education and Prevention Program. (1997). Expert Panel Report 2. *Guidelines for the diagnosis and management of asthma.* (NIH Publication No. 97-4051). Bethesda, MD: National Institutes of Health, National Heart, Lung and Blood Institute. Available online at www.nhlbi.nih.gov/guidelines/asthma/index.htm

Petronella, S. & Conboy-Ellis, K. (2003). Asthma epidemiology: Risk factors, case finding and the role of asthma coalitions. *Nursing Clinics of North America, 38*(4), 725-735.

U. S. Department of Health and Human Services. (2000). Respiratory diseases. In *Healthy People, 2010 Vol. 2* (2nd ed., pp 1-27). Washington, DC: U.S. Government Printing Office.

Weiss, KB. & Sullivan, SD. (2001). Health economics of asthma and rhinitis: Assessing the economic impact. *Journal of Allergy and Clinical Immunology, 107*(1), 3-8.

CHAPTER 2

PATHOPHYSIOLOGY OF ASTHMA

CHAPTER OBJECTIVE

Upon completion of this chapter the reader will recognize the impact of asthma as a chronic inflammatory disease on the role of the nurse when teaching patients the importance of anti-inflammatory medication for optimal asthma control.

LEARNING OBJECTIVES

After studying this chapter, the reader will be able to

1. recognize asthma as a chronic inflammatory disease of the airway.

2. identify three characteristics of asthma pathophysiology.

3. recognize five symptoms related to asthma pathophysiology.

4. explain the meaning of the term "airway remodeling."

5. state the importance of anti-inflammatory therapy for asthma control.

OVERVIEW

In light of the dramatic increase in asthma, as described in chapter 1, the National Heart, Lung, and Blood Institute (NHLBI) convened a national panel of asthma experts in the late 1980s. The goal of the panel was to make recommendations for the diagnosis and management of asthma based on sound scientific evidence. In-depth review of the science related to this disease has led to a redefinition of our understanding of asthma and the publication of the National Asthma Education and Prevention Program's (NAEPP's) Guidelines for the Diagnosis and Management of Asthma (1997). This chapter focuses on current understanding of the pathology of asthma based on the NAEPP's definition.

DEFINITION OF ASTHMA

The NAEPP issued its first expert panel report in 1991. Prior to 1991, asthma was defined as an acute disease with recurrent exacerbations. In response to accumulating scientific evidence, asthma was redefined as a chronic inflammatory disease that results in obstruction of the airways. This is an important distinction because the way we conceptualize the pathophysiology of asthma has major implications on treatment.

As research studies continued to expand knowledge, the expert panel reconvened and issued a second report (NAEPP, 1997) providing more scientific evidence of the role of inflammation in asthma. The report further described asthma as being characterized by episodes of airway obstruction that reversed spontaneously or with treatment. Inflammation was identified as the cause of airway hyperresponsiveness. Hyperresponsiveness, sometimes termed "twitchy" airways, is an important feature of asthma. Simply stated, hyperresponsiveness means that the airways narrow too easily and too much in response to many nonharmful stimuli (NAEPP, 1997).

An update to the guidelines was published in 2003 (National Asthma Education and Prevention Program [NAEPP] Expert Panel Report). This report provided further evidence of the role of inflammation and described the concept of remodeling as a result of chronic inflammation. Remodeling can be thought of as scarring, and it results in permanent airway damage. A large number of studies have investigated the concept of remodeling and the potential for early anti-inflammatory therapy to prevent permanent damage.

CHARACTERISTICS OF ASTHMA PATHOPHYSIOLOGY

Airway inflammation

Airway inflammation is categorized into two phases. The first, or acute phase, is immediate and short-lived. It involves bronchospasm with airway narrowing and responds readily to bronchodilator therapy. During the acute phase, cells that mediate the inflammatory response are recruited to the airway. Over several hours, these cells become activated and cause a persistent inflammation with a cycle of cell damage and repair (NAEPP, 1997). This second phase reaction, known as the late phase reaction, occurs 6 to 8 hours after the initial acute reaction. It manifests as a more severe reaction that is more difficult to treat.

The early-phase asthma reaction is depicted in Figure 2-1. The mast cell is the central feature in the initiation of the acute reaction. The mast cell contains many chemical inflammatory mediators.

FIGURE 2-1: EARLY-PHASE ASTHMA REACTION

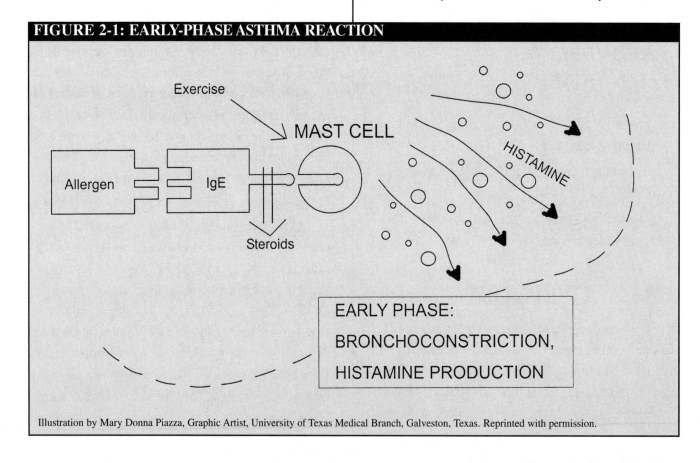

Exercise

MAST CELL

Allergen — IgE

HISTAMINE

Steroids

EARLY PHASE:

BRONCHOCONSTRICTION,

HISTAMINE PRODUCTION

Illustration by Mary Donna Piazza, Graphic Artist, University of Texas Medical Branch, Galveston, Texas. Reprinted with permission.

Activation of the mast cell by a trigger, such as tobacco smoke or an allergen, causes release of inflammatory mediators. Tobacco smoke acts directly on the mast cell and produces a short-lived response. Allergens, on the other hand, cause abnormal production of specific immunoglobulins, known as IgE, after the individual becomes sensitized to specific antigens. IgE creates a bridge between the antigen and mast cell. This bridging signals the release of many mediators, including histamine. IgE plays a critical role in asthma and higher levels are associated with more severe asthma (Busse, & Rosenwaller, 2003).

In response to the IgE mediated signal, airway smooth muscles rapidly contract (NHLBI/World Health Organization [WHO], 2003). Recent research indicates that smooth muscle mass also increases in size and may occupy as much as three times the normal area of the airway (Cohn, Elias, & Chupp, 2004).

Other mediators released by the mast cell include many powerful chemicals such as prostaglandins and leukotrienes that also act to constrict the airway. These chemicals send signals that result in recruitment of many other inflammatory agents to the airway. These agents stimulate each other in a process that is "redundant and self-perpetuating" (NHLBI/WHO, 2003).

Activation of mediators is illustrated in Figure 2-2. The mast cell is depicted as a powerful agent that spills its contents of mediators in several cascades. In addition to causing bronchoconstriction, these mediators cause small capillaries to leak, resulting in swelling, and stimulate mucus cells (NHLBI/WHO, 2003).

Activated mast cells recruit eosinophils to the airway. Eosinophils are leukocytes that are normally found in the blood. Their presence in the airway is an essential feature of asthma. Eosinophils con-

FIGURE 2-2: MAST CELL ACTIVATION

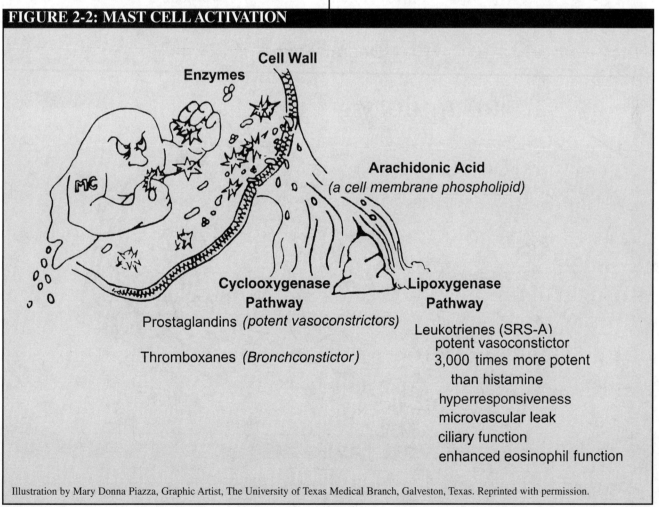

Illustration by Mary Donna Piazza, Graphic Artist, The University of Texas Medical Branch, Galveston, Texas. Reprinted with permission.

tain granules filled with many inflammatory agents; the most important of these agents is major basic protein. Figure 2-3 depicts the mast cell degranulating, or spilling its mediators and converting to a magnet. Eosinophils are chemically attracted to the airway by the pull of the activated mast cell. Eosinophils are depicted as warriors because of their destructive impact on the airway epithelium, which destroys epithelial cells leaving the airway wall denuded (NHLBI/WHO, 2003).

Figure 2-4 illustrates the effect of inflammatory mediators on the airway epithelium. Intact epithelium is critical for healthy functioning of the airways. Normally, the epithelium is lined with ciliated cells that act like an escalator to help increase mucus clearance. This layer of cells is destroyed as a result of chronic inflammation (NAEPP, 1997). Nerve endings become exposed and send repeated signals to constrict the airway.

Inflammation causes mucous glands to enlarge and increase in number (NAEPP, 1997). Mucus

FIGURE 2-3: ROLE OF EOSINOPHILS IN THE INFLAMMATORY PROCESS

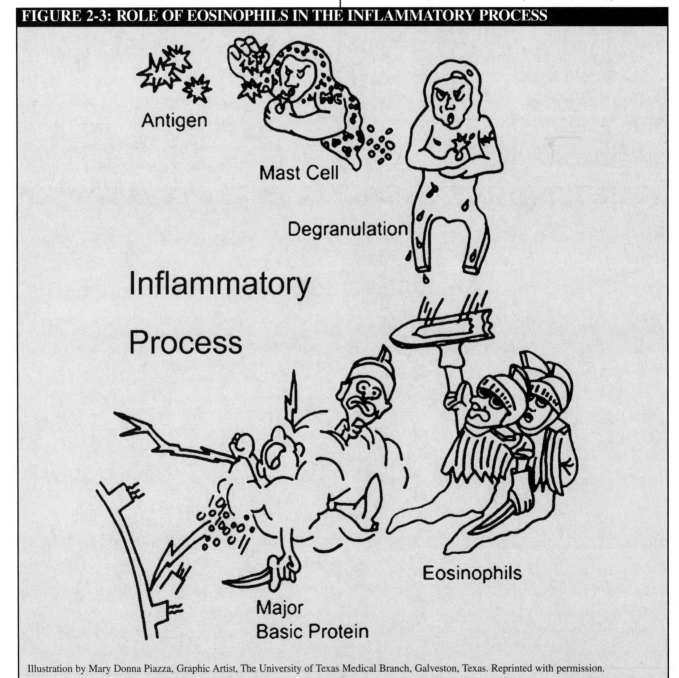

Illustration by Mary Donna Piazza, Graphic Artist, The University of Texas Medical Branch, Galveston, Texas. Reprinted with permission.

FIGURE 2-4: LOSS OF AIRWAY EPITHELIUM BY INFLAMMATORY MEDIATORS

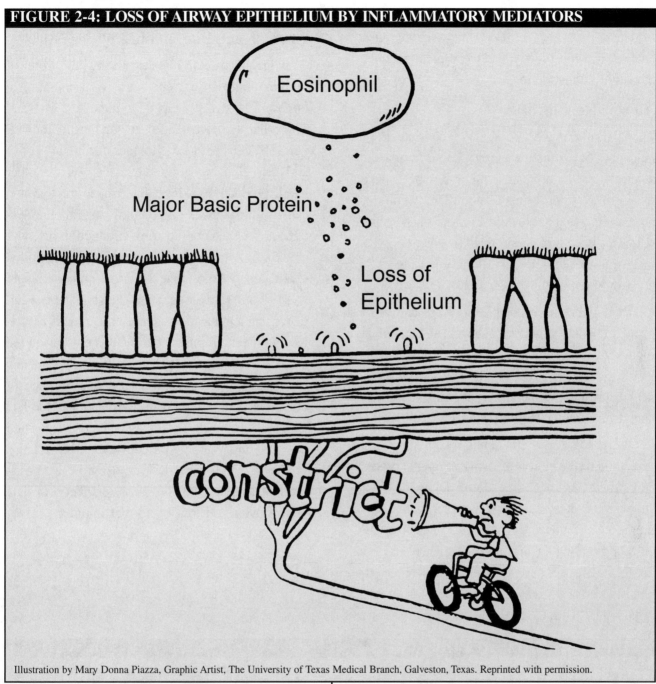

Illustration by Mary Donna Piazza, Graphic Artist, The University of Texas Medical Branch, Galveston, Texas. Reprinted with permission.

mixes with inflammatory cells and sloughed epithelial cells in the airway, creating mucus plugs and further obstruction (Cohn, Elias, & Chupp, 2004).

Infiltration of inflammatory cells into the airway also causes swelling and thickening of all airway layers. Thickening is an important feature of asthma because even modest thickening can cause severe airway narrowing. Thickening is correlated with obstruction and severity of disease. Inhaled corticosteroids (ICSs) have some effect on thickening; however, in those with long-standing asthma, ICS are less effective. It may be that permanent structural changes occur over time. In other words, asthma may not be completely reversible (Niimi, et al., 2004).

Asthma research over the past 15 years has focused on inflammation. As understanding of this process increases, it is becoming apparent that the inflammatory cell response in the airways varies from person to person. This may explain why some individuals respond differently to different asthma medications (Peters, 2003). Understanding these features will most likely lead to different treatment modalities in the future.

Airway Remodeling

Anti-inflammatory drugs are considered the mainstay of asthma therapy. These drugs can reverse some inflammatory processes, but it takes weeks to see improvement, and inflammation may not be completely resolved. Because of these persistent airflow limitations that do not respond to treatment, the definition of asthma now includes the concept of remodeling (NHLBI/WHO, 2003).

Remodeling is a complex process and is the result of many structural changes in the airway. Figure 2-5 depicts a simplified illustration of the end stage of this process. The airway thickening depicted results from collagen deposits beneath the denuded airway epithelium (NHLBI/WHO, 2003).

It is thought that remodeling is caused by long-term inflammation. It is an active, dynamic process that progresses over time. Remodeling has been shown to be present as early as age 9, with a slow progression from a reversible to an irreversible state, despite treatment. Unfortunately, there is no evidence, to date, that early use of ICSs will reduce the persistence of airway inflammation or prevent remodeling (Rasmussen, et al., 2002).

Airway Inflammation as a Loss of Normal Immune Balance

Current research is exploring the role of immune imbalance as a cause of asthma. Two opposing sets of T helper lymphocytes, Th1 and Th2 cells, are in a balanced state in healthy individuals. Th1 cells produce cytokines that are protective and help fight infection. Th2 cells, on the other hand, produce cytokines that are destructive and cause asthma and allergy. At birth, the immune system is imbalanced toward production of Th2 cytokines. After birth, Th1 cytokine production is stimulated by exposure to infections and, as a result, these systems are brought into balance. There is evidence that a reduced incidence of asthma is associated with certain infections, such as those acquired through exposure to other children in day care, and less frequent use of antibiotics. The absence of infections is associated with continuation of the Th2 pattern, thus the child with a genetic predisposition has the stage set to develop asthma or allergy. Further research is needed because it is also possible that asthma causes loss of regulation of Th1 lymphocytes and loss of normal immune balance (NHLBI/WHO, 2003).

FIGURE 2-5: AIRWAY REMODELING

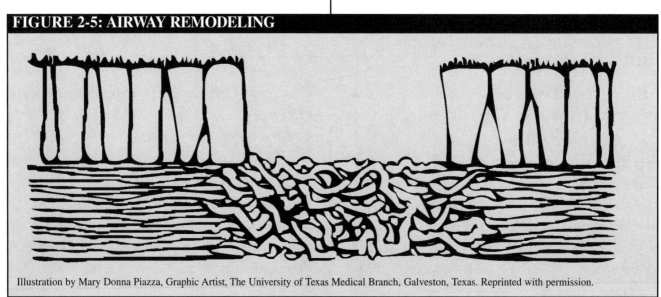

Illustration by Mary Donna Piazza, Graphic Artist, The University of Texas Medical Branch, Galveston, Texas. Reprinted with permission.

CLINICAL SIGNS AND SYMPTOMS

Asthma symptoms vary over time. Attacks can be sudden or gradual. Both sudden and gradual attacks can be severe in the absence of treatment. Inflammation is widespread throughout the airway and is responsible for clinical symptoms. Symptoms include recurrent episodes of wheezing, breathlessness, chest tightness, and coughing. Nocturnal cough, that is, cough in the middle of the night or early morning, or cough with exertion is especially characteristic of asthma (NHLBI/WHO, 2003). In fact, some individuals present with cough only and do not report history of wheezing. These individuals are said to have "cough variant asthma". Failure to recognize cough variant asthma leads to underdiagnosis of asthma and undertreatment.

Asthma symptoms are transient. They often increase or decease in relation to triggering events, such as seasonal exposure to pollen. Long periods of remission from symptoms may lead some individuals to accept symptoms and fail to seek treatment (NHLBI/WHO, 2003).

Wheezing is the most common symptom of asthma but it may be absent during severe asthma exacerbations. Absence of wheezing during severe attacks is a serious sign and indicates complete airway obstruction. Patients in this state have other signs such as cyanosis, difficulty speaking, and use of accessory muscles (NHLBI/WHO, 2003).

SUMMARY AND IMPLICATIONS FOR THERAPY

Asthma is a chronic inflammatory disease of the airway that produces bronchoconstriction, edema, and mucus formation. The inflammatory response is complex and self-perpetuating. Inflammatory events lead to airway obstruction and, over time, irreversible changes due to airway remodeling. Inflammation is persistent and widespread throughout the airway and produces characteristic asthma symptoms. Treatment must include anti-inflammatory therapy that is continuous and delivered throughout all parts of the airway. However, despite optimal treatment, some degree of lung damage is inevitable.

EXAM QUESTIONS

CHAPTER 2
Questions 7-11

7. Asthma can best be described as a disease that is

    a. acute and inflammatory.
    b. intermittent and obstructive.
    c. recurrent and obstructive.
    d. chronic and inflammatory.

8. The tendency of asthmatic airways to narrow excessively to common stimuli is called

    a. remodeling.
    b. vasoconstriction.
    c. hyperresponsiveness.
    d. bronchodilation.

9. Airway remodeling can best be described as

    a. permanent scarring.
    b. a static effect of the acute phase reaction.
    c. a response to acute inflammation.
    d. a temporary restructuring of the airway.

10. Symptoms of an acute attack produced by airway inflammation include

    a. hyperresponsiveness.
    b. cough in the early evening.
    c. tight sensation in the chest.
    d. cyanosis.

11. The impact of anti-inflammatory therapy in asthma is

    a. rapidly reduced inflammation.
    b. decreased inflammation over several weeks of therapy.
    c. elimination of the risk of remodeling.
    d. prevention of persistent inflammation.

REFERENCES

Busse, W. & Rosenwasser, L. (2003). Mechanism of asthma. *Journal of Asthma and Clinical Immunology, 111*, S799-804.

Cohn, L., Elias, J., & Chupp, G. (2004). Asthma: Mechanisms of disease persistence and progression. *Annual Review of Immunology, 22*, 789-815.

National Asthma Education and Prevention Program. (1997). Expert panel report 2. *Guidelines for the diagnosis and management of asthma.* (NIH Publication No. 97-4051). Bethesda, MD: National Institutes of Health, National Heart, Lung, and Blood Institute. Available online at www.nhlbi.nih.gov/guidelines/asthma/index.pdf

National Asthma Education and Prevention Program. (2003). Expert Panel Report: *Guidelines for the diagnosis and management of asthma: Update on selected topics 2002.* (NIH Publication No. 02-5074). Bethesda, MD: National Institutes of Health, National Heart, Lung and Blood Institute. Available online at http://www.nhlbi.nih.gov/guidelines/asthma/index.html

National Heart, Lung, and Blood Institute/World Health Organization. (2003). *Global initiative for asthma: Global strategies for asthma management and prevention.* (NIH Publication No. 02-3659). Retrieved September 12, 2002, from http://www.ginasthma.com

Niimi, A., Matusomoto, H., Amitani, R., Nakano, Y., Sakai, H., Takemura, M., et al. (2004). Effect of short-term treatment with inhaled corticosteroids on airway wall thickening in asthma. *American Journal of Medicine, 116*, 725-731.

Peters, S. (2003). Heterogeneity in the pathology and treatment of asthma. *American Journal of Medicine, 115*(3). Retrieved September 14, 2004, from http://home.mdconsult.com

Rasmussen, F., Taylor, D., Flannery, E., Cowan, J., Greene, J., Herbison, G., et al. (2002). Risk factors for airway remodeling in asthma manifested by a low post bronchodilator FEV1/vital capacity ratio. *American Journal of Respiratory and Critical Care Medicine, 165*, 1480-1488.

CHAPTER 3

DIAGNOSIS OF ASTHMA AND GOALS OF THERAPY

CHAPTER OBJECTIVE

Upon completion of this chapter, the reader will be able to recognize the diagnostic approach to asthma and the nurse's role in case finding.

LEARNING OBJECTIVES

After studying this chapter, the reader will be able to

1. identify five common clinical manifestations of asthma.

2. recognize the importance of the patient's history, the physical examination, and pulmonary function testing in diagnosing asthma.

3. recognize that asthma is classified according to severity level.

4. identify three characteristics of each severity level.

5. state four goals of asthma management.

6. identify the nurse's role in asthma case finding.

INTRODUCTION

The previous chapter focused on the pathophysiology of asthma. Airway inflammation and obstruction were described as producing characteristic symptoms associated with asthma. This chapter takes a more detailed look at symptoms from the perspective of the diagnostic process. A detailed history, a focused physical examination and pulmonary function testing are the most important tools in diagnosing asthma. Nurses must understand this process because they often play an important role in case finding.

CURRENT ISSUES IN THE DIAGNOSIS OF ASTHMA

Asthma is often underdiagnosed for various reasons. Most symptoms of asthma are nonspecific, resulting in a diagnosis of chronic bronchitis, wheezy bronchitis, recurrent pneumonia, gastroesophageal reflux, or recurrent upper respiratory infection (National Heart, Lung, and Blood Institute/World Health Organization [NHLBI/WHO], 2003). Patients contribute to the diagnostic problem because they often tolerate intermittent symptoms and young children are unable to perform pulmonary function maneuvers. In any event, improper labeling of the conditions leads to improper treatments such as antibiotics or cough medicine (NHLBI/WHO, 2003).

The issue of underdiagnosis has been the focus of efforts to improve asthma management by state asthma coalitions. These coalitions have identified other contributing factors such as reluctance of primary care providers to "label" a person with a chronic illness and fear that the diagnosis of asthma will prohibit the individual from joining the military or obtaining health insurance (Asthma Coalition of Texas, 2003).

Proper diagnosis is essential for proper treatment. This issue is so important that the Global Initiative for Asthma (NHLBI/WHO, 2003) has stated that the adage, "all that wheezes is not asthma," be more appropriately stated as "all that wheezes is asthma until proven otherwise."

THE ASTHMA HISTORY

People with asthma tend to be symptom free during the day, thus they are difficult to diagnose because they typically present with no symptoms during the office visit. The clinician must oftentimes rely heavily on the patient's history to establish the diagnosis. The history should be detailed and include the factors listed in Table 3-1.

TABLE 3-1: COMPONENTS OF THE ASTHMA HISTORY

- Family history of asthma or allergy
- History of atopic dermatitis or allergic rhinitis
- Symptoms, frequency, and pattern of occurrence
- Triggers
- Exercise tolerance
- Cough, especially at night
- Hospitalizations, urgent care, or emergency room visits
- Medications, response to medications, and frequency of use
- Seasonal worsening of symptoms

(NAEPP, 1997)

Asthma is partly under genetic control. A history in one or both parents is highly predictive of asthma. Asthma is also an allergic disease. The presence of other allergic diseases, such as allergic rhinitis or atopic dermatitis (eczema), are predictive of asthma. However, it should be remembered that some individuals with no family history of allergic disease do have asthma.

Asthma symptoms include wheezing, shortness of breath, cough, tight chest, and large swings (variability) in peak flow readings. Some people do not experience wheezing, but rather complain of cough. For reasons that are not completely understood, cough usually occurs in the middle of the night. The healthcare provider should ask specifically about nighttime cough between the hours of 1:00 or 2:00 a.m. to 6:00 a.m. The lowest point in diurnal variation of airflow occurs during these hours and this factor partially explains increase in nighttime cough.

The healthcare provider should ask about the pattern, frequency, and duration of symptoms as well as the association of such symptoms with particular triggering events. Symptoms are often seasonal. Many individuals report increase in symptoms during the fall and winter months. A history of episodic symptoms is highly suggestive of asthma.

The history should also obtain information about the patient's response to triggers, specifically if symptoms worsen in the presence of triggers. Question about triggers such as smoking by self or others in the home and the presence of pets in the house. Exercise requires careful consideration. Many people with asthma experience shortness of breath after approximately 10 minutes of exercise that resolves with a rest period. The patient commonly interprets this as being "out of shape."

Despite hospitalizations and emergency room (ER) visits, the patient may not have received the correct diagnostic label. The patient who has visited the ER commonly describes improvement of symptoms after receiving an albuterol treatment. This response indicates reversal of airway obstruction and is highly suggestive of asthma.

The patient should be asked about use of medications, frequency of use, and effect of medications on symptoms. Commonly, patients borrow rescue medication from other family members or purchase epinephrine inhalers (marketed as Primatine or Bronchaid Mist) over the counter. These are unsafe practices and need to be discouraged. Nevertheless, frequency of rescue medication use is helpful in assessing asthma severity.

THE PHYSICAL EXAMINATION

The physical examination focuses on the chest, upper respiratory tract, and skin. Because asthma symptoms are variable, the examination may be completely normal; however, the most common finding is wheezing upon auscultation. Air trapping and prolonged exhalation are also features of asthma. Hyperexpansion of the chest may be noted; and if asthma has been long-standing, the individual may have a barrel chest.

Most children and some adults with asthma also have allergic symptoms. These include continuous clear, watery nasal drainage; pale nasal mucosa; itchy eyes, nose and throat; and sneezing. Venous congestion due to nasal swelling leads to "allergic shiners" or dark circles under the eyes. Children may deny an itchy nose, but parents confirm the "allergic salute"—rubbing of the nose in an upward motion. Frequent itching can result in a horizontal crease across the bridge of the nose. Thick, discolored mucus usually indicates sinusitis.

In children, the skin is assessed for atopic dermatitis. During infancy, the atopic rash can occur all over the body except the diaper area, but usually is seen on the cheeks and progresses to the extremities. In children, the lesions are predominately seen in the flexural creases of the arms and legs (Fireman & Slavin, 1996). Atopic dermatitis usually resolves in the school-age years, but it can continue into adulthood.

PULMONARY FUNCTION TESTING

The history and physical alone are not reliable in assessing the degree of airway obstruction (NAEPP, 1997). As an objective measure, pulmonary function testing is necessary in diagnosing asthma. Pulmonary function is measured by spirometry. In the past, spirometry was cumbersome, highly technical, expensive, and limited to specialty clinics. Technical innovations have led to widespread use of compact, inexpensive spirometers in primary care.

Because of their importance and common use, the nurse should have a basic understanding of spirometry. Nurses can relate to the importance of objective assessment because they have a long history of monitoring blood pressure for hypertension or blood sugar for diabetes. The role of spirometry in the care of persons with asthma is analogous to monitoring blood pressure or blood sugar in persons with hypertension or diabetes.

A spirometer measures the volume of inspired and expired air over time. In asthma, the focus of testing is on expired air. The patient is instructed to take a maximal inhalation and blow long and hard into a mouthpiece attached to a computerized spirometer. Results of the maneuver are displayed numerically and graphically. A trained expert examines the results for patterns of airway obstruction. Frequently, obstruction is identified by pulmonary function testing despite a normal physical examination and denial of dyspnea by the patient. This is precisely the reason why pulmonary function testing is essential. Patients and physicians often underestimate the degree of airway obstruction.

In most people with asthma, airway obstruction is reversible. Baseline pulmonary function testing is repeated after administration of an albuterol challenge (administration of albuterol, followed by repeat pulmonary function testing to see if the medication caused at least 12% or greater improvement). Demonstration of 12% or greater improvement in forced expiratory volume in 1 second (FEV_1), an important measure of pulmonary function, indicates reversibility and, combined with the history and physical, establishes the diagnosis. Spirometry is also used to monitor response to asthma therapy over time.

CLASSIFICATION OF ASTHMA SEVERITY

Asthma varies in severity from individual to individual. After the diagnosis is established, the next step is to determine the severity of the asthma. The National Asthma Education and Prevention Program (NAEPP, 1997) established definitions of asthma severity, which have since been further refined (NHLBI/WHO, 2003). See Table 3-2.

Classification levels have been shown to relate to varying degrees of inflammation. This system is important because therapy is initiated according to degree of inflammation or severity level. Assignment of severity level is based upon clinical features before treatment. Symptoms are rarely a perfect match for a particular category level. The patient should be assigned the highest category that is consistent with his clinical presentation. Severity can change over time so it is reassessed with each patient visit. When asthma control is achieved, a person with severe persistent asthma should have only mild intermittent symptoms. However, those with mild asthma can have a severe acute exacerbation.

TABLE 3-2: CLASSIFICATION OF ASTHMA SEVERITY BY CLINICAL FEATURES BEFORE TREATMENT

Step	Symptoms	Pulmonary Function
I. Mild Intermittent	Less than two times per week Brief exacerbations Nocturnal symptoms less than twice per month	Forced expiratory volume in 1 second (FEV_1) (FEV_1) > 80% predicted or peak expiratory flow (PEF) > 80% of personal best. PEF or FEV_1 variability < 20%
II. Mild Persistent	Twice per week, but less than once per day Exacerbations may affect activity and sleep. Nocturnal symptoms more than twice per month	FEV_1 > 80% predicted or PEF > 80% of personal best. PEF or FEV_1 variability 20%-30%
III. Moderate Persistent	Daily symptoms Exacerbations may affect activity and sleep. Nocturnal symptoms more than once per week Daily use of short-acting beta$_2$-agonist	FEV_1 > 60%-< 80% predicted or PEF 60%-80% of personal best. PEF or FEV1 variability > 30%
IV. Severe Persistent	Continual symptoms Frequent exacerbations Frequent nocturnal symptoms Limitation of physical activity	FEV_1 > 60% predicted or PEF > 60% of personal best. PEF or FEV1 variability > 30%

Note. From National Asthma Education and Prevention Program. (1997). Expert panel report 2. *Guidelines for the diagnosis and management of asthma.* (NIH Publication No. 97-4051). Bethesda, MD: National Institutes of Health, National Heart, Lung, and Blood Institute. Available online at www.nhlbi.gov/guidelines/asthma/asthgdln.pdf

GOALS OF ASTHMA THERAPY

The National Asthma Education and Prevention Program established these goals of asthma therapy (NAEPP, 1997):

- Prevent symptoms.

- Minimize the need for hospitalizations and emergency visits.

- Minimize missed school or work days.

- Provide optimal pharmacotherapy with minimal side effects.

- Achieve near normal pulmonary function.

- Maintain normal activity levels, including participation in sports.

- Meet patient's and family's expectation of satisfaction with care.

Asthma goals serve as a guide to therapy and patient education. Goals are slightly modified for the older adult and the pregnant woman with asthma. These modifications will be addressed in later chapters.

THE NURSE'S ROLE IN CASE FINDING

As discussed in chapter 1, asthma is a major public health problem, and efforts are being initiated to address asthma on this level. Efforts include improved case finding to identify persons with undiagnosed asthma in order to provide proper treatment and lessen the burden of asthma morbidity. Most of the prevalence data available are based on subjective patient responses to telephone surveys. Although helpful, these data are not highly accurate.

In an effort to increase accuracy, case finding approaches are becoming popular. One effort being used in Texas is school-based surveillance among elementary school children (Petronella & Conboy-

Ellis, 2003). The standard school health intake form has been modified to include several broad-based questions about respiratory problems. Spirometry is performed on children older than age 7 to validate the responses. In a related project, high school athletes were screened for asthma via spirometry. Surprisingly, 20% of the students tested had below normal pulmonary function results (Brooks & Hayden, 2003).

School nurses often provide feedback that students frequently suffer asthma-like symptoms but lack health data in their records. School nurses as well as nurses in any setting can assist with case finding. Table 3-3 lists questions that can be asked to help determine a diagnosis of asthma. A positive response to any of these questions is sufficient reason for the nurse to recommend referral for diagnostic testing.

TABLE 3-3: QUESTIONS TO CONSIDER IN THE DIAGNOSIS OF ASTHMA

1. Have you had an attack or recurrent attacks of wheezing?

2. Do you have a troublesome cough at night?

3. Do you wheeze or cough after exercise?

4. Do you wheeze, cough, or have chest tightness after exposure to airborne allergens or pollutants?

5. Do your colds "go to the chest" or take more than 10 days to clear up?

6. Do your symptoms improve with appropriate anti-asthma treatment?

(NHLBI/WHO, 2003)

SUMMARY

Asthma is often undiagnosed or misdiagnosed for various reasons. Proper diagnosis is critical for proper treatment. Diagnosis is established by obtaining and interpreting a detailed asthma history, and performing a focused physical examination and pulmonary function testing. The diagnostic process includes classifying the severity of asthma to provide a basis for therapy. Asthma management goals guide therapy and patient and family education. Nurses need to understand the diagnostic process and related issues as part of their role in case finding across.

CASE STUDY

The school nurse observes that each day when the pollen count is high, John, age 10, is in the clinic complaining of shortness of breath. She reviews his health history but finds nothing significant. She also notices that he has a clear, runny nose and that he sneezes and itches his eyes. He appears tired, so she asks if he is getting enough sleep. He responds affirmatively but complains of waking in the middle of the night with a troublesome cough.

Answer the following study questions, writing your responses on a separate sheet of paper. Compare your responses with the answers provided.

1) What signs and symptoms lead you to suspect that John is suffering from asthma?

2) What treatment options are available to the school nurse to help John?

3) What are three additional questions you could ask John to help confirm your suspicion of asthma?

4) What is the most appropriate course of action for the school nurse?

Answers to Case Study

1) Symptoms that suggest asthma include the seasonal nature of the symptoms, the presence of allergy symptoms (sneezing; clear, runny nose; and itching) and nocturnal cough.

2) The school nurse has no treatment options because there is no documentation that John has asthma, nor does he have any asthma medications available.

3) Additional questions that the nurse can ask John

include:

a. Have you been to the emergency room in the last year for breathing problems?

b. Does your mother or father have asthma or allergies?

c. Do you wheeze or cough after running?

4) The most appropriate course of action for the school nurse is to talk to John's parents and explain the need to have John's breathing difficulty evaluated.

EXAM QUESTIONS

CHAPTER 3
Questions 12-16

12. A common symptom of asthma is

    a. nighttime cough.

    b. dark circles under the eyes.

    c. rash in the flexor creases of the arms and legs.

    d. barrel chest.

13. The most objective tool to establish an accurate diagnosis of asthma is

    a. a detailed history.

    b. a focused physical examination.

    c. spirometry.

    d. a chest x-ray.

14. John has daily wheezing, PEF 70% of personal best, a nighttime cough three times per week, and he refuses to play sports because of difficulty breathing. He receives an asthma severity classification of

    a. mild intermittent.

    b. mild persistent.

    c. moderate persistent.

    d. severe persistent.

15. Asthma management goals include

    a. proper diagnostic labeling.

    b. minimal use of medications.

    c. few missed school or work days.

    d. monitoring with spirometry.

16. The nurse's role in case finding includes

    a. becoming proficient in spirometry.

    b. securing detailed asthma histories.

    c. assessing presence of wheezing and prolonged expiration.

    d. referring persons with common asthma symptoms for evaluation.

29

REFERENCES

Asthma Coalition of Texas. (2003). Unpublished conference summary. September, 2003. Austin, Texas.

Brooks, E. & Hayden, ML. (2003). Exercise-induced asthma. *The Nursing Clinics of North America, 38*, 689-696.

Fireman, P. & Slavin, R. (1996). *Atlas of Allergies* (2nd ed.). London: Mosby-Wolfe.

National Asthma Education and Prevention Program. (1997). Expert panel report 2. *Guidelines for the diagnosis and management of asthma.* (NIH Publication No. 97-4051). Bethesda, MD: National Institutes of Health, National Heart, Lung, and Blood Institute. Available online at www.nhlbi.nih.gov/guidelines/asthma/index.pdf

National Heart, Lung, and Blood Institute/World Health Organization. (2003). *Global initiative for asthma: Global strategies for asthma management and prevention.* (NIH Publication No. 02-3659). Retrieved September 12, 2002, from http://www.ginasthma.com

Petronella, S. & Conboy-Ellis, K. (2003). Asthma epidemiology: Risk factors, case finding, and the role of asthma coalitions. *The Nursing Clinics of North America, 38*, 725-735.

CHAPTER 4

MONITORING
SIGNS AND SYMPTOMS OF ASTHMA

CHAPTER OBJECTIVE

Upon completion of this chapter, the reader will be able to recognize the role of symptom and peak flow monitoring in the management of asthma.

LEARNING OBJECTIVES

After studying this chapter, the reader will be able to

1. state the importance of educating patients to recognize early warning signs.

2. identify patients who may benefit from use of symptom diaries.

3. recognize the usefulness of peak flow monitoring in asthma management.

4. state what is meant by the term "personal best."

5. interpret peak flow readings using the zone concept.

6. identify actions to take when peak flow is in the yellow or red zone.

7. provide patient education on symptom and peak flow monitoring.

OVERVIEW

The nature of asthma as a self-perpetuating and redundant inflammatory disease demands that symptom-based treatment be started as early as possible.

Initial symptoms, usually referred to as early warning signs, indicate to the patient and caregiver that therapy needs adjusting to prevent a severe exacerbation. Failure to recognize early symptoms leads to asthma that is difficult to treat and high rates of acute healthcare utilization. This chapter focuses on recognition of early warning signs, symptom and peak flow monitoring, and the nurse's role in educating the patient regarding asthma monitoring.

EARLY WARNING SIGNS

Early warning signs are experienced before the start of an asthma attack. Common early warning signs include: allergy symptoms (itching; sneezing; clear, runny nose), decreased exercise tolerance, drop in peak flow reading, fatigue, moodiness, and headache. These signs vary among individuals and may vary from episode to episode in the same individual. Although not classified as an early warning sign by the National Asthma Education and Prevention Program, upper respiratory tract infections (URIs) trigger asthma exacerbations, and typically URI-induced attacks are severe. Because signs of a cold often precede a severe attack, patients do well to consider a URI an early warning sign and begin adjusting their dose of long-term controller medication.

Extensive work with school-age children in an asthma camp setting reveals that children tend to ignore early warning signs (Meng & McConnell,

2002) because they wish to be like other healthy children. Symptoms are a reminder that the child with asthma is different, and furthermore, symptoms interfere with activities that are important to the child. However, ignoring early warning signs leads to symptoms that are difficult to manage. Teaching children to be aware of early warning signs and to report them to an adult is one of the most challenging topics in asthma education.

Most of the literature on symptom recognition focuses on those with asthma who cannot perceive airway obstruction, the so-called "poor perceivers." Some poor perceivers overestimate asthma symptoms. This is a problem because it leads to excessive use of medication and healthcare services. Underestimation of symptoms is more common and is estimated to affect 15% to 75% of patients with asthma, usually males. It is by far the more significant clinical problem and has been linked to the fatality prone profile; a list of criteria that help identify patients who are at risk for asthma-related death. Underestimation of symptoms causes delays in seeking treatment, underuse of controller medication, and avoidable deaths. Poor perception of asthma symptoms is more common in persons with long-standing asthma and is thought to be an adaptation response, perhaps similar to adaptation experienced by patients suffering from chronic pain. Persons with poor perception of airway obstruction need an objective tool such as a peak flow meter to guide self-management decisions (Meng & McConnell, 2003).

SYMPTOM DIARIES

Symptom diaries provide the patient and family with a method of self-assessment at home. Key symptoms to be monitored should be included in the diary. Table 4-1 provides an example of a symptom diary.

Diaries are designed to be completed on a daily basis, but not all groups of patients will be inclined to dedicate time to daily recording. Adherence may improve if the healthcare provider recommends using diaries at critical times for the patient, such as during troublesome seasons or at the first sign of a URI. Interest and feedback from the nurse will further increase the likelihood that diaries are completed.

Parents of infants and young children are commonly anxious and distressed during periods of breathlessness, especially because young children cannot identify symptoms. This group, in particular, may find the use of a symptom diary reassuring. Diaries may also be useful for the short-term in patients whose asthma is not yet under control, in patients who are monitoring the effect of new treatments, and in patients who are trying to identify environmental or occupational triggers that make their asthma worse.

PEAK FLOW MONITORING

Definition

Peak flow is the largest flow rate that can be exhaled after taking a maximal inhalation. It is a measure of airway obstruction. Peak expiratory flow rate (PEFR) is one of the pulmonary function parameters measured by spirometry, but can also be measured by small, inexpensive handheld meters. The focus of this discussion is on the handheld method.

Handheld peak flow meters are simple, easy to use, and the results are reproducible. These characteristics make peak flow recording feasible as a self-management tool for home use. Peak flow is effort dependent; that is, the patient must generate a hard, fast exhalation for an accurate reading. For this reason, the patient's technique needs to be carefully taught and monitored over time in order to obtain consistent and reliable results.

Uses of Peak Flow

Peak flow meters are designed for monitoring symptoms. They are not diagnostic tools. Properly used, they offer several benefits, namely:

TABLE 4-1: EXAMPLE OF PATIENT SYMPTOM DIARY

	Symptoms				Treatment		Peak Flow		Comments
Date	Wheeze	Cough	Activity	Sleep	Beta$_2$-agonist	Inhaled steroid	AM	PM	

Wheeze:	none = 0; some = 1; medium = 2; severe = 3
Cough:	none = 0; occasional = 1; frequent = 2; continuous = 3
Activity:	normal = 0; can run short distance or climb three flights of stairs = 1; can walk only = 2; missed school or work or stayed indoors = 3
Sleep:	fine = 0; slept well, slight cough = 1; awake two to three times with cough or wheeze = 2; bad night, awake most of time = 3

Note. Adapted from National Asthma Education and Prevention Program. (1997). Expert Panel Report 2. *Guidelines for the diagnosis and management of asthma.* (NIH Publication No. 97- 4051). Bethesda, MD: National Institutes of Health, National Heart, Lung, and Blood Institute. Available online at www.nhlbi.nih.gov/guidelines/asthma/asthgdln.pdf

- Detecting airway obstruction before symptoms appear

- Monitoring response to treatment for asthma exacerbations

- Indicating whether emergency care is needed

- Monitoring response to changes in drug therapy

- Identifying asthma triggers

Adherence to daily peak flow monitoring and recording is notoriously poor. As with symptom diaries, peak flow adherence can be improved if it is used during times of greatest vulnerability for the patient and if the provider gives the patient feedback. Peak flow is not recommended for all patients. Those with mild asthma do not benefit from peak flow monitoring, but patients with moderate to severe persistent asthma should have peak flow meters available and use them during exacerbations or when therapy is changing. Minority and poor children have shown greater improvement in asthma severity than white children when using peak flow as part of the management plan (Yoos, Kitzman, McMullen, Henderson, & Sidora, 2002).

Currently, peak flow is considered a more sensitive indicator of airway obstruction than appearance of early warning signs; however, this belief is being challenged. In a study that compared use of peak flow to symptom-based management plans, school children with stable asthma responded to changes in symptoms by increasing their controller medication when peak flow readings were normal. In this particular study, peak flow did not enhance asthma management, even during acute exacerbations (Wensley & Silverman, 2004). Although peak flow monitoring is recommended by the National Asthma Education and Prevention Program (NAEPP) guidelines (1997), many clinicians have begun to question the usefulness of recommending peak flow monitoring for all patients with stable asthma. Certainly, persons with severe asthma and persons who have poor perception of airway obstruction can benefit from peak flow monitoring.

The NAEPP update (2003) recommends either symptom based monitoring or peak flow monitoring as equally effective. This expert panel notes that peak flow monitoring in patients with moderate or severe asthma enhances patient-clinician communication and increases patient awareness and control of their disease.

Technique

Several different brands of peak flow meters are on the market. Readings may vary among different brands of meters, so the nurse should instruct the patient to use one brand consistently. Young children are developmentally unable to perform the peak flow technique. Generally, children ages 5 and older are capable of performing peak flow. A suggested rule of thumb in assessing peak flow readiness is to determine if the child can blow out candles on a birthday cake. Table 4-2 lists peak flow technique.

TABLE 4-2: PEAK FLOW TECHNIQUE
1. Move the indicator to the bottom of the scale.
2. Stand up.
3. Take a deep breath, filling lungs completely.
4. Seal your lips around the mouthpiece. Do not put your tongue in the hole.
5. Blow out as hard and fast as you can.
6. Write down the number you get.
7. Repeat steps 1-5 two more times and record the highest number in your log.
(NAEPP, 1997)

Unpublished data from video analyses of children attending an asthma day camp indicated that the most frequent technique errors made by children were failure to stand up and failure to take a big breath (Meng, 1998). Children did benefit from repeated instruction and continuous coaching on proper technique.

Personal Best

Personal best is the highest number that the patient can achieve during a 2- to 3-week period when asthma is well controlled (when there are no symptoms). Although there are predicted norms for peak flow based on age, gender, and height, each person's best peak flow is individual and may be higher or lower than predicted. It is important for individuals to determine their own "best" and to set this as a goal in their self-management plan.

To determine personal best, peak flow is monitored twice per day, in the morning and 10 to 12 hours later. If a beta$_2$-agonist is used, the reading should be taken before and after using the beta$_2$-agonist. The peak flow maneuver is repeated three times at each reading and the highest of the three attempts is recorded. Results are recorded for a 2- to 3-week asymptomatic period. The highest number is the individual's personal best. Some people are unable to achieve a personal best that is near the expected normative value. A short course of oral steroids may be needed to establish personal best in these cases.

Peak flow is based on height. Therefore, personal best in growing children changes over time, similar to changing clothes size. The same procedure described above is used to reset an individual's personal best after periods of growth.

The Zone Concept

After the personal best is determined, peak flow zones can be calculated. Zones provide a method of interpreting the peak flow results. Readings fall into good, moderate, or poor categories.

Zones must be meaningful to patients. A symbol that is universally understood is the traffic light. People understand that a green light means "go," yellow means "slow down," and red means "stop." This traffic light analogy is built into the zone concept.

When a person is at or within 80% of personal best, he is in the green zone. The recommended action is to, "go," or proceed with usual activities

with no adjustment to the management plan. A reading between 80% and 50% of personal best falls into the yellow zone. Yellow zone readings mean that the person's asthma may not be under optimal day-to-day control; the person should "slow down" and take action. Symptoms may not be evident when readings fall near the top of the yellow zone, yet the reading indicates some degree of obstruction. The person should follow instructions from their personal management plan (see chapter 13) for medication adjustments. Peak flow readings of 50% or below personal best signal a medical emergency. The person should "stop" activities and take immediate action. Instructions in the red zone are to take rescue medication right away and call the healthcare provider.

Ideally, peak flow is recorded twice per day. Twice daily recordings allow the provider to assess diurnal variation. Morning and afternoon readings that are within 20% of each other are indicators of good control. Diurnal variability greater than 20% indicates loss of asthma control and signals the need to adjust controller therapy (NAEPP, 1997). Some persons are unable to monitor twice per day. In such cases, early morning readings are preferred.

THE NURSE'S ROLE IN EDUCATING THE PATIENT

Asthma, by nature, is variable. People with asthma need to have a self-monitoring plan in place for early detection of deteriorating control.

The nurse should review early warning signs with all patients. Some individuals may become frustrated when questioned about their early warning signs because they are sometimes difficult to identify. The nurse should reassure the patient that by asking these questions, they will become more focused on making the appropriate observation in the future.

The nurse should help school-age children understand the importance of telling an adult when they recognize symptoms. This intervention may include helping the child identify appropriate adults to tell when they are at school. Children who are reluctant to identify symptoms can sometimes be motivated by linking early recognition and treatment to improved performance in activities such as sports or band.

Monitoring should be linked to an action in the self-management plan. When providing education, the nurse should consider individual needs and abilities to perceive symptoms in planning the nature and intensity of monitoring. As mentioned previously, some groups may benefit from symptom diaries and peak flow meter monitoring.

Consideration must also be given to availability of peak flow meters. Although inexpensive relative to spirometry, families with limited income may find the cost prohibitive, especially when a second meter is needed at school. The nurse should assess barriers to accessing equipment and explore creative means to overcome barriers. Peak flow prices may be lower at durable medical equipment stores than at pharmacies, and some insurance companies may support the purchase if a prescription is provided. Pharmaceutical companies may sometimes donate meters to a clinic. Children who attend asthma camps may be given peak flow meters as part of the educational program.

Regardless of the symptom monitoring method chosen, the nurse must provide regular assessment and feedback to the patient and family. If peak flow meters are used, the technique needs to be evaluated and corrected, if needed, at every visit.

SUMMARY

Recognition of early warning signs and symptom monitoring is critical for optimal asthma control. Patients and families may have different needs, perceptual abilities, and preferences regarding the type of monitoring used. The nurse needs to consider these differences in planning education.

Patients with severe asthma and with poor perceptual ability benefit from peak flow monitoring and regular feedback. Symptom monitoring needs to be linked to actions in the individual's self-management plan.

CASE STUDY

Paul, age 18, is a first-year college student. He is on the college football team. He has had moderate persistent asthma since he was age 4. His asthma is troublesome during the fall and winter. Each fall for the past 3 years he has had an emergency room visit because he could not sense that his asthma was flaring up. He wants to do well on the football team, so has come to the clinic to see if there are any new asthma medications that will better control his asthma.

Answer the following study questions, writing your responses on a separate sheet of paper. Compare your responses with the answers located at the end of the chapter.

1. What symptom monitoring strategy will most likely benefit Paul?

2. Is Paul likely to benefit from education about recognizing early warning signs?

3. What strategies can the nurse use to increase the likelihood that Paul will adhere to symptom monitoring?

4. How can the nurse help Paul set management goals based on symptom monitoring?

Answers to Case Study

1. Paul would benefit from peak flow monitoring. He cannot rely on subjective recognition of symptoms. Peak flow is an objective and reliable measure of airway obstruction.

2. Paul does not have the ability to sense his early warning signs. He fits the definition of a person with poor perception of airway obstruction. Because his asthma is long-standing, he has probably adapted to poor pulmonary function. However, as Paul starts to monitor his peak flow, he may benefit from reflecting on a feeling of tight chest or other symptoms when his peak flow reading is low. He could also be instructed to guess his peak flow reading, measure the actual peak flow, and compare the differences. Over time, he may develop more accuracy in estimating the degree of his airway obstruction.

3. The nurse can increase adherence by stressing the importance of measuring peak flow during Paul's asthma season—fall and winter. The nurse can also link peak flow and early treatment to improved performance in football and provide consistent feedback at each visit.

4. Paul needs to be instructed on the proper technique for determining his personal best. His highest reading during a 2- to 3-week period of optimal asthma control is his personal best. His personal best becomes his goal for self-management.

EXAM QUESTIONS

CHAPTER 4
Questions 17-23

17. Recognition of early warning signs of an asthma attack is important because these signs

    a. give the patient extra time to plan a visit to the emergency room.

    b. indicate the need to stay home and rest.

    c. alert the patient to begin early treatment.

    d. ensure prevention of a severe attack.

18. Patients who may benefit from symptom diaries include

    a. adolescents with busy school schedules.

    b. parents of toddlers.

    c. adults with known triggers.

    d. patients on a stable medication program.

19. Peak flow is best described as the

    a. largest inhalation a person can take.

    b. fastest breath taken.

    c. largest amount of air exhaled.

    d. fastest inhalation and exhalation.

20. Peak flow monitoring is most useful in people

    a. with mild intermittent asthma.

    b. with mild persistent asthma.

    c. ages 3 to 7.

    d. who cannot detect signs of airway obstruction.

21. Personal best describes

    a. the best asthma control possible.

    b. the best peak flow effort despite symptoms.

    c. consistent readings in the green zone for 2-3 weeks.

    d. the highest peak flow number with no symptoms during a 2- to 3-week period.

22. John's personal best peak flow is 300 but measures 125 today. John's current peak flow zone is

    a. green.

    b. top of the yellow.

    c. bottom of the yellow.

    d. red.

23. The nurse should advise John to

    a. take rescue medication and call the physician immediately.

    b. re-measure his peak flow.

    c. stay home and rest.

    d. go to the emergency room.

REFERENCES

Meng, A. & McConnell, S. (2002). Decision-making in children with asthma and their parents. *Journal of the American Academy of Nurse Practitioners, 14*, 363-371.

Meng, A. & McConnell, S. (2003). Symptom perception and respiratory sensation: Clinical implications. *Nursing Clinics of North America. 38*:4, 737-748.

Meng, A. (1998). Videotape analysis of peak flow technique in school age children attending an asthma day camp. Unpublished data. Galveston, Texas.

National Asthma Education and Prevention Program. (1997). Expert panel report 2. *Guidelines for the diagnosis and management of asthma.* (NIH Publication No. 97-4051). Bethesda, MD: National Institutes of Health, National Heart, Lung, and Blood Institute. Available online at www.nhlbi.nih.gov/guidelines/asthma/index.pdf

National Asthma Education and Prevention Program. (2003). Expert Panel Report: *Guidelines for the diagnosis and management of asthma: Update on selected topics 2002.* (NIH Publication No. 02-5074). Bethesda, MD: National Institutes of Health, National Heart, Lung and Blood Institute. Available online at http://www.nhlbi.nih.gov/guidelines/asthma/index.html

Wensley, D. & Silverman, M. (2004). Peak flow monitoring for guided self-management in childhood asthma. *American Journal of Respiratory and Critical Care Medicine, 170*, 606-612.

Yoos, H., Kitzman, H, McMullen, A., Henderson, C., & Sidora, K. (2002). Symptom monitoring in childhood asthma: A randomized clinical trial comparing peak expiratory flow rate with symptom monitoring. *Annals of Allergy, Asthma, & Immunology, 88*(3), 283-291.

CHAPTER 5

PHARMACOLOGIC MANAGEMENT OF ASTHMA

CHAPTER OBJECTIVE

Upon completion of this chapter, the reader will be able to identify the role of quick-relief and long-term controller medications in the management of asthma and provide patient and family education related to optimal use of asthma medications.

LEARNING OBJECTIVES

After studying this chapter, the reader will be able to

1. identify the role of quick-relief medication in the treatment of asthma.

2. recognize three classes of quick-relief medications.

3. identify the role of long-term controller medications in the treatment of asthma.

4. recognize three classes of long-term controller medications.

5. recognize side effects of asthma medications.

6. recognize the stepwise approach to medication therapy based on asthma severity levels.

7. identify correct techniques for medication administration.

8. provide patient education on use of asthma medications.

OVERVIEW

Asthma is a chronic disease with no cure, but it is controllable. The previous chapter discussed assessment, that is, recognition of early warning signs and symptom monitoring. This chapter focuses on general pharmacologic interventions for managing asthma. Asthma medicines are used to prevent and control symptoms, to reduce the frequency and severity of acute attacks, and reverse acute airflow obstruction. Asthma medicines are grouped into two general classes: quick-relief ("rescue") or long-term controller medications. Persons with persistent asthma need both classes of medications. Pharmacologic interventions for emergency room (ER) care and specific groups, such as children, the childbearing woman, and the older adult, will be discussed in later chapters.

QUICK-RELIEF MEDICATIONS

Quick-relief medications are used for immediate relief of acute bronchoconstriction and its related symptoms (cough, wheeze and tight chest). These drugs include short-acting $beta_2$-agonists, anticholinergics, and oral corticosteroids.

Short-Acting Beta$_2$-Agonists

Short-acting inhaled $beta_2$-agonists, or "rescue medications," are the drugs of choice for relief of acute, episodic symptoms and for pretreatment of exercise-induced asthma. These drugs relax constricted airway smooth muscles and promote mucus clearance. They can relieve symptoms within 15 to 20 minutes, and have a duration of action of 4 to 6 hours. Inhaled beta$_2$-agonists provide more rapid relief with fewer symptoms than oral beta$_2$-agonists. Although commonly prescribed in the past, oral beta$_2$-agonists are no longer listed as a treatment option in the National Asthma Education and Prevention Program's guidelines (2003).

Quick-relief inhaled beta$_2$-agonists include albuterol, pirbuterol, bitolterol, and levalbuterol (R-albuterol). Of these drugs, albuterol is the most commonly prescribed. Dosages and routes of administration of quick-relief medications are listed in Table 5-1.

Side effects of beta$_2$-agonists include tachycardia, skeletal muscle tremor, and hypokalemia. Parents of young children often report hyperactivity as a troublesome side effect of albuterol. Over time, tolerance to side effects usually develops; however,

TABLE 5-1: COMMON QUICK-RELIEF BRONCHODILATORS, DOSAGES, AND DOSAGE FORMS

Medication	Form	Adult Dose	Child Dose
Beta$_2$-agonists			
Albuterol	**Metered-dose inhaler** **(*MDI*)** 90 mcg/puff 200 puffs/canister	2 puffs 5 minutes before exercise 2 puffs 3–4 times/day prn	1–2 puffs 5 minutes before exercise 2 puffs 3–4 times/day prn
Albuterol	*Nebulizer Solution* 5 mg/mL (0.5%) 2.5 mg/mL 1.25 mg/3 mL 0.63 mg/3 mL	1.25 mg in 3 cc of saline q 4–8 hours*	0.05 mg/kg (minimum 1.25 mg, maximum 2.5 mg) in 3 cc of saline q 4–6 hours*
		* May double dose for severe exacerbation	
Levalbuterol	0.31 mg/3 mL 0.63 mg/3 mL 1.25 mg/3 mL	0.63 mg–2.5 mg q 4–8 hours	0.025 mg/kg (minimum 0.63 mg, maximum 1.25 mg) q 4–8 hours
Anticholinergics			
Ipratropium	***MDI*** 18 mcg/puff 200 puffs/canister	2-3 puffs q 6 hours	1-2 puffs q 6 hours
	Nebulizer Solution 0.25 mg/mL (0.025%)	0.25 mg q 6 hours	0.25-0.5 mg q 6 hours
Systemic Corticosteroids			
Prednisone	1, 2.5, 5, 10, 20, 50 mg tablets; 5 mg/cc, 5 mg/5 cc oral solution	short "burst" 40-60 mg/day or divided in two doses for 3-10 days	short "burst" 1-2 mg/kg/day maximum 60 mg/day for 3-10 days

Note. Adapted from National Asthma Education and Prevention Program. (2003). Expert Panel Report. *Guidelines for the diagnosis and management of asthma: Update on selected topics 2002.* (NIH Publication No. 02-5074). Bethesda, MD: National Institutes of Health, National Heart, Lung and Blood Institute. Available online at http://www.nhlbi.nih.gov/guidelines/asthma/index.htm

some individuals do not develop tolerance. Levalbuterol may be an option for these individuals. Levalbuterol is an isomer of albuterol that has the therapeutic action of its parent drug with none of the side effects. Although expensive, levalbuterol is often more acceptable to patients than albuterol. Unfortunately, levalbuterol is only available as a nebulized solution.

In the past, practitioners frequently prescribed quick-relief beta$_2$-agonists for regular, around the clock use. This practice is no longer recommended because regular use of beta$_2$-agonists does not adequately control asthma. In fact, frequent or increased use of quick-relief beta$_2$-agonists is a warning signal that asthma control is deteriorating and such use is associated with increased risk of death. Overuse of quick-relief beta$_2$-agonists may result in failure of therapeutic response when it is most needed—during an acute attack. Generally, use of more than two canisters per year of quick-relief beta$_2$-agonists is considered excessive use and indicates the need to reevaluate and increase long-term controller therapy.

Oral Corticosteroids

Onset of action of oral corticosteroids is slow (4 to 6 hours). Nevertheless, these drugs are classified as quick relief because they speed recovery in moderate to severe exacerbations, prevent relapses, and decrease ER visits. Corticosteroids target inflammatory mediators in multiple ways. Their actions result in decreased activation and recruitment of inflammatory cells into the airway. They also enhance the function of beta$_2$-receptors (DeKorte, 2003).

A short course (3 to 10 days, depending on severity of exacerbation) of therapy is prescribed for severe acute exacerbations. A typical dose is prednisone 1 to 2 mg to a maximum of 60 mg per day, for 5 to 10 days. There is no need to taper the dose with short-course dosing, and side effects are generally not experienced with short-course therapy.

Anticholinergic Agents

Inhaled anticholinergic agents (such as ipratropium bromide) are bronchodilators, but they do not effect the airway smooth muscle in the same manner as beta$_2$-agonists. Anticholinergics reduce vagal cholinergic tone to the airways and block bronchoconstriction caused by inhaled irritants. They have no effect on airway inflammation. They are not as potent as the beta$_2$-agonists and have a slower onset of action (30 to 60 minutes).

Anticholinergics are useful in persons who have a diminished response to beta$_2$-agonists. They are generally used in adults but can also be used in children. Anticholinergics are often given in combination with nebulized beta$_2$-agonists because of their additive effect on bronchodilation. Anticholinergics may also be used as the bronchodilator of choice in those who experience tachycardia and arrhythmia from quick-relief beta$_2$-agonists. Side effects associated with anticholinergics are minimal, mainly bitter taste and dry mouth.

LONG-TERM CONTROLLER MEDICATIONS

Inhaled Corticosteroids

Corticosteroids are the most potent and consistently effective medications for the long-term control of asthma. Corticosteroids suppress airway inflammation, decrease hyperresponsiveness (the tendency of the airways to respond to stimuli by constricting), control symptoms and improve pulmonary function. Inhaled corticosteroids (ICSs) have been the mainstay of therapy for prevention of irreversible loss of lung function. Used properly, that is, continuously on a daily basis, ICSs reduce exacerbations, hospital admissions, and asthma-related deaths (DeKorte, 2003) and are the preferred treatment for patients with persistent asthma at all severity levels.

A number of different ICSs are available. Table 5-2 lists commonly used ICSs as well as other controller medications.

ICSs differ in potency and bioavailability. Bioavailability is an important factor to consider in drug selection. Unique chemical properties of each drug affect their ability to be absorbed into the systemic circulation (bioavailability). Systemic absorption is associated with increased side effects, so in the case of ICSs, bioavailability is not desirable. Newer ICSs, such as fluticasone and budesonide, are less bioavailable than the older ICSs, triamcinolone

TABLE 5-2: COMMON ASTHMA CONTROLLER MEDICATIONS

Medication	Dose Form	Adult Dose	Child Dose
Combination			
Fluticasone/Salmeterol (Advair)	DPI 100 mcg, 250 mcg, or 500 mcg/ 50 mcg	1 inhalation bid; dose depends on severity	1 inhalation bid; dose depends on severity
Inhaled Corticosteroids			
Beclomethasone CFC (Qvar)	Metered-dose inhaler (MDI), 42 or 84 mcg/puff	168-504 mcg Low 504-840 mcg Medium > 840 mcg High	84-336 mcg Low 336-672 mcg Medium > 672 mcg High
Beclomethasone HFA	MDI, 40 or 80 mcg/ puff	80-240 mcg Low 240-480 mcg Medium > 480 mcg High	80-160 mcg Low 160-320 mcg Medium > 320 mcg High
Budesonide *Entocort EC*	Dry-powdered inhaler (DPI), 200 mcg/inhalation	200-600 mcg Low 600-1,200 mcg Medium > 1,200 mcg High	200-400 mcg Low 400-800 mcg Medium > 800 mcg High
Inhalation suspension for nebulization (child dose)	0.25 mg respule 0.5 mg respule		0.5 mg Low 1.0 mg Medium 2.0 mg High
Fluticasone *Flovent*	MDI, 44, 110, 220 mcg/puff	88-264 mcg Low 264-660 mcg Medium > 660 mcg High	88-176 mcg Low 176-440 mcg Medium > 440 mcg High
	DPI, 50, 100 or 250 mcg/inhalation	100-300 mcg Low 300-600 mcg Medium > 600 mcg High	100-200 mcg Low 200-400 mcg Medium > 400 mcg High
Leukotriene Modifiers			
Montelukast	4 or 5 mg chewable tablet 10 mg tablet	10 mg qhs	4 mg qhs (ages 2-5) 5 mg qhs (ages 6-14) 10 mg qhs (ages >14)
Zafirlukast	10 or 20 mg tablet	40 mg qd or 20 mg bid	20 mg qd (ages 7-11) or 10 mg bid
Zileuton	300 or 600 mg tablet	2,400 mg qd in four divided doses	

Note. Adapted from National Asthma Education and Prevention Program. (2003). Expert Panel Report. *Guidelines for the diagnosis and management of asthma: Update on selected topics 2002.* (NIH Publication No. 02-5074). Bethesda, MD: National Institutes of Health, National Heart, Lung and Blood Institute. Available online at http://www.nhlbi.nih.gov/guidelines/asthma/index.htm

and beclomethasone. Fluticasone and budesonide are therefore more available to the target organ—the lung. New ICSs are currently being designed with even less bioavailability than fluticasone.

Local side effects of ICSs include hoarseness, occasional cough, and candidiasis (thrush). These side effects are well controlled with the use of a spacer and by rinsing and spitting after dose administration. All presently available ICSs are bioavailable, so there are systemic effects with each depending on the drug dose, potency, and ability of the drug to be absorbed from the lung. Spacers increase drug delivery to the lung rather than the stomach, so use of spacers decreases bioavailability. Long-term treatment with high doses of ICSs may be associated with skin thinning, easy bruising, adrenal suppression and decreased bone density. The clinical significance of these effects is not yet known, but there is concern that long-term cumulative effects of ICSs may increase the risk of osteoporosis and glaucoma (DeKorte, 2003).

Although the search for the ideal ICS with no side effects continues, some progress has been made. New metered-dose preparations of ICSs are formulated with hydrofluoroalkane (HFA), a propellant with decreased particle size that allows for deeper drug penetration in the lung. Because penetration is better than with the older chlorofluorocarbon (CFC) formulations, HFA formulations allow for reduced dosing by as much as 50% (DeKorte, 2003). These formulations can be identified by the "HFA" on the canister label and shape of the mouthpiece. The CFC mouthpiece is oval and the HFA mouthpiece is round. Healthcare practitioners are advised to carefully read the medication insert of the new HFA inhalers. For bronchodilators, the doses from CFC and HFA inhalers appear to be equivalent, but for some ICSs, the HFA preparation delivers a greater amount of smaller particles to the lung, resulting in greater efficacy but more systemic effects (National Heart, Lung, and Blood Institute [NHLBI]/World Health Organization [WHO], 2003).

The ICS dosage depends on asthma severity; higher dosages are used for more severe asthma. Current therapy is based on the fact that at high levels, ICSs have a flat dose/response curve. In other words, at higher dosage levels, increasing the dosage produces no further benefit, but does increase the risk of side effects. Current recommendations (National Asthma Education and Prevention Program [NAEPP], 2003) call for add-on therapy with another class of controller medication rather than increasing the dosage of the ICS.

ICSs are commonly underprescribed by providers and their use is poorly adhered to by patients. Surveys indicate that only two thirds of patients with severe persistent asthma have been prescribed an ICS and of those with an ICS, only half adhere to their plan (DeKorte, 2003). This means that only one third of patients are adequately treated with long-term controller medication. Strategies to increase adherence include reducing dosing frequency by prescribing higher concentrations of the drug and assessing patient preference for type of delivery system.

Long-Acting Beta$_2$-Agonists

Long-acting beta$_2$-agonists (LABs) include salmeterol and formoterol. Their duration of action is longer than 12 hours but decreases somewhat with long-term use. Mechanism of action of the LABs is the same as with the quick-relief beta$_2$-agonists, but over time LABs may have a small anti-inflammatory effect as well. Used as an adjunct to ICS therapy, LABs should always be used in combination with an ICS. The addition of a LAB to ICS therapy provides a synergistic effect that is more effective than doubling the dose of an ICS alone. Patients receiving combination therapy have demonstrated improvements in pulmonary function, decreased nocturnal symptoms, better control of exercise-induced asthma, and less reliance on rescue medication.

Better asthma control from combination therapy has led to the development of two-in-one inhalers, such as Advair (fluticasone plus salmeterol). Fixed combination inhalers have several advantages: (a) increased adherence to treatment plan by patients, (b) assurance that the LAB is always administered with the ICS, and (c) reduced cost. One drawback of the two-in-one inhaler is that it does not allow for increasing the ICS dose when there is an asthma flare up. Because high doses of LABs may cause arrhythmias, patients are taught not to increase doses with the combination drug. An additional inhaler containing only inhaled corticosteroid may be prescribed to allow for increasing the ICS dose in the case of worsening asthma.

Leukotriene Modifiers

The leukotriene modifiers are a class of drugs that became available in 1996. They include leukotriene-receptor antagonists (zafirlukast and montelukast) and a leukotriene synthesis inhibitor (zileuton). The former are approved in children. The advantage of the leukotrienes is that they are taken orally; therefore, they have increased acceptance with patients.

The leukotrienes are less potent medications than ICSs and are not substitutes for ICS therapy. They are recommended as add-on therapy for patients with mild to moderate persistent asthma to allow for reduction of the ICS dose. New recommendations include the use of montelukast for children as young as age 2 because of improvement in pulmonary function. However, montelukast is not as effective as moderate dose of budesonide in preventing exercise-induced symptoms (NHLBI/ WHO, 2003).

Leukotrienes are less effective than LABs as add-on therapy; however, surveys indicate that they are being used beyond current NAEPP guideline recommendations. Adult patients with severe asthma report using leukotrienes as combination therapy, even though the efficacy of leukotrienes

for severe asthma has not been established (Snyder, Blanc, Katz, Yelin, & Eisner, 2004). Leukotrienes are well tolerated with few side effects, but zileuton is associated with liver toxicity. Monitoring of liver function tests is recommended with zileuton therapy.

Other Controller Medication Options

The nonsteroidal anti-inflammatory medications, cromolyn sodium and nedocromil, are options for management of asthma. Cromolyn and nedocromil are very safe with almost no side effects; however, they are much less potent than the ICSs and have the disadvantage of requiring dosing three or four times daily. For these reasons, use of nonsteroidal anti-inflammatory medication is declining.

Theophylline is also a treatment option. Theophylline, a methylxanthine, has bronchodilator and some anti-inflammatory activity but is not as effective as quick-relief bronchodilator or ICS medications. Theophylline has many drug interactions and side effects. It also has a narrow therapeutic range, requiring frequent invasive monitoring to determine blood serum levels. Use of theophylline is declining because of these disadvantages.

ANTI-IgE ANTIBODY

Currently, there is interest in monoclonal antibodies for treatment of asthma. Although these drugs were developed in the 1970s, their application to asthma is new. Many of these drugs are still in research investigations and will be available to clinical practice in the near future. Basically, the monoclonal antibodies target various inflammatory mediators, such as immunoglobulin (Ig)E or the interleukins, to block the inflammatory cascade.

Anti-IgE antibody (omalizumab) is a recombinant humanized, monoclonal antibody that is currently available for clinical use. Anti-IgE binds to the same region of the IgE molecule that interacts with the IgE receptor, thus blocking the allergic cascade (Bousquet, Wenzel, Holgate, Lumry, Freeman, & Fox, 2004). Persons with very severe, difficult to treat asthma, benefit from anti-IgE. It is used as add-on therapy to ICS and may allow for reduced ICS dosing.

Omalizumab is administered subcutaneously and reaches peak serum concentrations in 3 to 14 days. The dose is determined by the patient's baseline IgE level and body weight. Frequency of administration is every 2 to 4 weeks for a minimum of 12 weeks. Omalizumab appears to be safe but side effects include fatigue and musculoskeletal, digestive, and urtricarial skin reactions (DeKorte,

2003). The drug is expensive and is reserved for severe asthma.

STEPWISE APPROACH TO ASTHMA THERAPY

Selection of asthma medications and dosing are based on asthma severity level. The NAEPP guidelines (2003) identify four severity levels, as presented in chapter 3. Table 5-3 lists recommended treatment according to severity level.

Severity level is established before treatment, and the patient is assigned to the highest severity

TABLE 5-3: THE STEPWISE APPROACH TO MANAGING ASTHMA			
Severity Level	**Symptoms/Day** **Symptoms/Night**	**Peak Flow Variability**	**Daily Medications**
Step 4 Severe Persistent	continual daily frequent night	$\leq 60\%$ $> 30\%$	Preferred treatment: High-dose ICS AND long-acting inhaled beta$_2$-agonists, AND, if needed, systemic corticosteroids (2mg/kg/day, generally not to exceed 60 mg/day)
Step 3 Moderate Persistent	daily > 1 night/week	> 60%–< 80% > 30%	Preferred treatment: Low to medium dose ICS and LAB Alternative: Medium dose ICS OR low to medium dose ICS and leukotriene modifier or theophylline
Step 2 Mild Persistent	>2/week but< 1x/day > 2 nights/month	$\geq 80\%$ 20%-30%	Preferred treatment: Low-dose ICS Alternative Treatment: Cromolyn, leukotriene modifier, nedocromil or sustained-release theophylline to serum concentration of 5–15 mcg/mL
Step 1 Mild	< 2 days/week $\leq$ 2 nights/month	$\geq 80\%$ < 20%	No daily medication needed Short-course systemic corticosteroids for severe exacerbations

Note. Adapted from National Asthma Education and Prevention Program. (2003). Expert Panel Report. *Guidelines for the diagnosis and management of asthma: Update on selected topics 2002.* (NIH Publication No. 02-5074). Bethesda, MD: National Institutes of Health, National Heart, Lung and Blood Institute. Available online at http://www.nhlbi.nih.gov/guidelines/asthma/index.htm

level consistent with the patient's history, symptoms, physical findings, and pulmonary function. The stepwise plan is used as a guide to designing therapy because other considerations such as cost and availability of treatment need to be taken into consideration. The patient's response to therapy needs to be continually monitored to determine effectiveness of medications and the plan needs to be adjusted because individuals' asthma severity can change over time.

Patients at all severity levels need access to quick-relief bronchodilators. Patients with persistent asthma need long-term controller medication in addition to quick-relief bronchodilator therapy. Two approaches to long-term controller dosing are acceptable. A dose consistent with the patient's severity level can be initiated and increased if optimal control is needed. On the other hand, maximal dosing can be initiated at the onset to gain rapid control of symptoms followed by gradually stepping down the dose. Many clinicians prefer the latter approach because adherence to daily controller therapy is poor. Response to therapy may take weeks and failure to see immediate improvement is discouraging to patients. Initial maximal dosing helps the patient appreciate the benefits of controller therapy because control is achieved sooner.

When sustained control is achieved with absolutely no symptoms, a reduction in controller therapy to a lower step is carefully considered. Sustained control may take 3 months or longer to achieve. Monitoring is continued even after control is achieved because asthma severity continually changes.

PREVENTION

Patients with moderate to severe asthma should be advised to receive the influenza vaccine each year. Inactivated influenza vaccine is safe to administer to adults and children, including those with severe asthma (NHLBI/WHO, 2003).

TECHNIQUES OF MEDICATION ADMINISTRATION

Great improvements have been made in asthma medications. They are highly effective, but only if administered correctly. It is not uncommon to see treatment failures despite appropriate medication plans. Depending on the device and the patient's inhalation technique, 20% to 80% of the dose may never reach the lung because it is swallowed (DeKorte, 2003). Patients must be taught correct administration techniques and the nurse must evaluate technique at every visit. Asthma medications are available as metered-dose inhalers (MDIs), dry powdered inhalers (DPIs), or nebulized solutions. Each formulation requires a different administration technique.

Metered-Dose Inhalers and Spacers

The MDI is the most common device used to take asthma medication. The MDI allows the patient to inhale a specific amount of medicine (a "metered dose") in an aerosol form. The device consists of a metal canister, which keeps the medicine under pressure, and a plastic sleeve, which helps to release the medication. When the canister is pressed, or "actuated," medicine particles are propelled toward the throat and inhaled. Proper MDI technique is critical. Incorrect technique results in deposition of medication on the oral mucosa. The medication is then swallowed and delivered to the stomach. The effect on the lungs is minimal.

See Table 5-4 for MDI technique.

MDI spacers, sometimes called "holding chambers," are strongly encouraged for people of all ages because they deliver medication more effectively to the lungs and reduce side effects. Spacers hold the puff of medicine in a chamber between the MDI canister and the patient. Spacers eliminate the need to coordinate inhalation and exhalation with canister actuation. When the patient uses the spacer, slow

TABLE 5-4: METERED-DOSE INHALER ADMINISTRATION TECHNIQUES
1. Remove the cap and hold the inhaler upright.
2. Insert the inhaler into spacer.
3. Remove the spacer mouthpiece.
4. Shake the inhaler/spacer.
5. Actuate the inhaler to release the medication.
6. Exhale fully, then take a slow, deep breath over 3 to 5 seconds.
7. Hold your breath for 10 seconds to allow the medicine to reach deeply into lungs.
8. Repeat puff as directed, waiting 1 minute between puffs.
(NAEPP, 1997)

inhalation results in delivery of the medication to the lungs. Spacers are supplied with mouth pieces and various-sized face masks for infants and young children, or anyone who has difficulty maintaining a good lip seal on the mouthpiece.

Spacers should always be used with MDIs, regardless of age. An additional advantage of using spacers to deliver medication to the lungs is that less drug is deposited in the stomach where it can become bioavailable. Decreasing bioavailability decreases side effects. Spacers also decrease the side effects of thrush and cough.

Dry Powdered Inhalers

Several asthma medications are available as DPIs. An advantage of the DPIs is that no spacer is required. A disadvantage of the DPIs is that each medication is actuated by a technique unique to that particular drug. It is important to review the manufacturer's administration directions for each DPI.

In-Check Dial™

The In-Check Dial™ is a new handheld device that enables the practitioner to measure the force of the patient's inhalation. Inspiratory force is an important measure because different inhalers require a certain amount of force to release the med-

ication. The patient is instructed to take a maximal inhalation by breathing in through the In-Check Dial™ mouthpiece. The inspiratory force generated moves the In-Check Dial™ marker along a calibrated scale. The marker reading is compared to a chart listing inspiratory forces required to actuate inhalers from different manufacturers.

Sometimes patients are unable to generate sufficient force to release the medication. Patients may benefit from training, but often the medication of choice has to be changed to a different formulation that requires less inspiratory force.

THE NURSE'S ROLE IN EDUCATING THE PATIENT

Nurses have an important role in educating patients about proper use of asthma medications. From the patient point of view, recommending use of asthma medications is illogical and contradicts past experience. Most people take medication because a symptom is bothersome or threatens well-being. Relief is expected soon after taking the medication or else the medication is considered ineffective. Common experiences for most people include using medications to relieve pain, fever, or acute infection. If the patient applies this logic to asthma therapy, quick-relief beta$_2$-agonists would be used daily and long-term controller medication would be reserved for acute exacerbations. In fact, this pattern of drug use is often seen in clinical practice.

Correct use of asthma medication is inconsistent with the patient's past medication experience. Patients are taught that quick-relief medication (i.e., medication that "works") is used sparingly and that long-term controller medication (medication that doesn't work right away) is taken on a daily basis, even when symptoms are not present. The nurse must explore patients' perceptions and expectations of medication and dispel unrealistic expectations. Set the expectation that ICSs do "work" if taken as directed.

The nurse needs to spend time explaining inflammatory changes in the airway and the relationship of asthma medications to these changes. These are difficult concepts and patients learn them best when concrete models or illustrations are used. Repeat teaching at intervals and reinforce correct medication use with positive reinforcement.

The importance of correct technique cannot be understated. The nurse should assess the patient's inhalation ability and technique and reinforce correct technique at every visit.

SUMMARY

Two classes of asthma medications, quick-relief bronchodilators and long-term controllers, were reviewed in light of asthma severity classification levels. ICSs are the mainstay of asthma therapy but are no longer recommended in high doses. The preferred treatment for severe asthma is the addition of LABs to low or medium dose ICS therapy. Inhaled medication must be administered using spacers and proper technique. Patient adherence to ICSs is typically poor. The nurse plays a critical role in educating the patient regarding optimal medication therapy.

CASE STUDY

Carol, a 21-year-old college student, had moderate persistent asthma as a school-age child. She believes that she outgrew her asthma and no longer has medication on hand. Winter used to be her worst season, and this winter she has experienced a return of symptoms that have bothered her for the past 5 weeks. She complains of daily cough and awakens with cough two times per week. She comes to the clinic to request a quick-relief inhaler. She has no difficulty taking a sufficiently deep inspiration to use inhalers effectively, but she has limited financial resources.

Answer the following study questions, writing your responses on a separate sheet of paper. Compare your responses with the answers located at the end of the chapter.

1. What is Carol's current asthma severity classification?

2. What is the preferred medication treatment for Carol?

3. Because Carol is 21-years-old and has limited financial resources, should a spacer be recommended?

4. What pattern of medication adherence might Carol be likely to adapt?

5. What teaching concepts should the nurse stress to increase medication adherence?

Answers to Case Study

1. Based on the presence of daily symptoms and twice weekly nocturnal symptoms, Carol is classified with moderate persistent asthma.

2. The preferred treatment for Carol is a low to medium dose ICS with an LAB such as Advair. A typical dose would be Advair 250/50 bid. This dose provides 500 mcg of fluticasone per day, which is a medium ICS dose. In addition, Carol needs a quick-relief beta$_2$-agonist, such as albuterol, 2 puffs every 4 to 6 hours, as needed for acute symptoms.

3. Carol will need a spacer to properly administer the albuterol. If it is not feasible for her to invest in a spacer, consideration can be given to the use of pirbuterol, which is supplied with an autoinhaler. Another option is to teach the patient to use a cardboard tube, such as an empty toilet paper roll, as a spacer.

4. Carol is a high risk for suboptimal medication adherence for several reasons. She believes that she has outgrown her asthma, she is requesting quick-relief medication, and she has limited financial resources.

5. The nurse should elicit Carol's treatment expec-
    tations and correct misconceptions. In addition,
    the nurse needs to use pictures or models to
    carefully review the action of medications and
    how each medication works in the airway. The
    nurse should give Carol a definite message that
    Advair is an extremely effective medication if
    taken as directed. The nurse must also teach
    correct medication technique so that the benefit
    of the medication is experienced.

EXAM QUESTIONS

CHAPTER 5
Questions 24-30

24. Rapid acting beta$_2$-agonists, such as albuterol are used in asthma therapy

    a. to prevent severity of asthma attacks.

    b. to reduce severity of attacks.

    c. as a post exercise treatment.

    d. as quick relief treatment for acute symptoms.

25. Quick-relief asthma medications include

    a. prednisone.

    b. salmeterol.

    c. anti-IgE.

    d. theophylline.

26. The most effective long-term controller medications are

    a. long-acting bronchodilators.

    b. nonsteroidal anti-inflammatory agents.

    c. inhaled corticosteroids.

    d. leukotriene modifiers.

27. Common side effects of ICS therapy include

    a. liver damage.

    b. irritability.

    c. thrush.

    d. bad taste.

28. Monotherapy with low-dose ICSs are the preferred therapy for persons with an asthma severity rating of

    a. mild intermittent.

    b. mild persistent.

    c. moderate persistent.

    d. severe persistent.

29. The nurse assesses the patient's MDI technique as correct when the patient inhales over

    a. 1 to 2 seconds.

    b. 3-5 seconds.

    c. 6-8 seconds

    d. 9-10 seconds.

30. The most important concept to stress when providing medication education to the patient with asthma is

    a. patients at each severity level need controller medication.

    b. ICSs should be changed if they fail to work right away.

    c. it is safe to take quick-relief bronchodilators as often as needed.

    d. ICSs are effective if taken every day.

REFERENCES

Bousquet, J., Wenzel, S., Holgate, S., Lumry, W., Freeman, P., & Fox, H. (2004). Predicting response to omalizumab, an anti-IgE antibody, in patients with allergic asthma. *Chest, 125*, 1378-1386.

DeKorte, C. (2003). Current and emerging therapies for the management of chronic inflammation in asthma. *American Journal of Health System Pharmacists, 60*, 1949-1961.

National Asthma Education and Prevention Program. (1997). Expert panel report 2. *Guidelines for the diagnosis and management of asthma.* (NIH Publication No. 97-4051). Bethesda, MD: National Institutes of Health, National Heart, Lung, and Blood Institute. Available online at www.nhlbi.nih.gov/guidelines/asthma/index.pdf

National Asthma Education and Prevention Program. (2003). Expert Panel Report: *Guidelines for the diagnosis and management of asthma: Update on selected topics 2002.* (NIH Publication No. 02-5074). Bethesda, MD: National Institutes of Health, National Heart, Lung and Blood Institute. Available online at http://www.nhlbi.nih.gov/guidelines/asthma/index.html

National Heart, Lung, and Blood Institute/World Health Organization. (2003). *Global initiative for asthma: Global strategies for asthma management and prevention.* (NIH Publication No. 02-3659). Retrieved September 12, 2002, from http://www.ginasthma.com

Snyder, L., Blanc, P., Katz, P., Yelin, E., & Eisner, M. (2004). Leukotriene modifier use and asthma severity: How is a new medication being used by adults with asthma? *Archives of Internal Medicine, 164*, 617-622.

CHAPTER 6

ENVIRONMENTAL CONTROL OF ASTHMA

CHAPTER OBJECTIVE

Upon completion of this chapter, the reader will be able to recognize common asthma triggers and provide education regarding basic environmental control to patients and families.

LEARNING OBJECTIVES

After studying this chapter, the reader will be able to

1. recognize the gene-environment connection to the development of asthma symptoms.

2. state the difference between irritants and allergens as asthma triggers.

3. identify seven common asthma triggers.

4. state the importance of controlling asthma triggers in the home.

5. recognize five strategies to control environmental triggers.

6. provide patient education on trigger management.

OVERVIEW

The previous chapter discussed the role of medication in the treatment of asthma. Although extremely important, pharmacotherapy is only one aspect of asthma management. Avoidance of triggers is the most effective step in controlling asthma because triggers are the cause of airway inflammation and symptoms in sensitized persons. The most important triggers are inhaled allergens. For optimal control of asthma, the patient must incorporate environmental control measures into the treatment plan. The nurse has an important role in assisting patients and families to identify and avoid asthma triggers.

GENE–ENVIRONMENT INTERACTION

Asthma has an important genetic component. Expression of asthma and sensitization to asthma triggers are under genetic influence and vary among individuals. Currently, asthma is thought of as a diverse group of related conditions that require multiple genes for expression of clinical symptoms. The presence of certain genes predisposes individuals to become sensitized to particular allergens after repeated exposure. This is an area of intense research investigation but at the present time is not well understood (Board of Health Promotion and Disease Prevention [HPDP] & Institute of Medicine [IOM], 2004).

The nurse should recognize that people with asthma vary in their response to allergens. Allergens that trigger symptoms in one individual with asthma may not trigger symptoms in another person with asthma. Acquired allergen sensitivity is a function of duration and frequency of exposure. That is, the longer the person with a genetic predisposition is exposed to high doses of allergen, the more likely he is to become sensitized to that allergen.

IRRITANTS AND ALLERGENS

Asthma triggers are classified as irritants or allergens. Irritants cause bronchoconstriction and produce a less severe asthmatic response than allergens. Common irritants are tobacco smoke and indoor and outdoor pollution such as ozone, fumes, and aerosol sprays. Most persons with asthma react to irritants. Allergens on the other hand, produce airway inflammation and cause more severe exacerbations of asthma. Allergens are only problematic to persons who become sensitized to a particular allergen. Common inhaled allergens are dust mites, animal dander, cockroach allergen, indoor fungi (mold), and outdoor pollens.

TRIGGERS IN THE HOME

Control of asthma triggers has focused on indoor strategies for several reasons. Indoor allergens have increased in developed countries where homes have been insulated for energy efficiency. Use of wall-to-wall carpet, heating, cooling, and humidification provide ideal habitats for dust mites, cockroaches, insects, mold, and bacteria. Better methods of sealing and failure to ventilate homes prevent air exchange, which increases the load of indoor pollutants (National Heart, Lung, and Blood Institute/ World Health Organization [NHLBI/WHO], 2003). More time is being spent indoors than in the past, increasing duration of exposure to indoor allergens. A recent study concluded that exposure to indoor allergens leads to more severe asthma and decreased pulmonary function in sensitized persons (Langley, et al., 2003). Finally, although control strategies are almost impossible to apply outdoors, they can be applied indoors. The majority of time within the home is spent in the bedroom, so special emphasis is given to controlling triggers in the bedroom.

Dust Mites

Dust mites are ubiquitous in the United States except in high, arid altitudes, so most people with asthma are sensitized to dust mites. Mites feed off of human scales and are found in highest concentrations in bedding. They are also found in carpet and soft furnishings. Carpets are a possible source of reinfestation of bedding (NHLBI/WHO, 2003). Humidity is essential for growth of mites, so keeping humidity below 50% is important. Dust removal with a damp cloth is essential. Other recommended measures for controlling dust mites are listed in Table 6-1.

TABLE 6-1: MEASURES FOR REDUCING EXPOSURE TO DUST MITE ALLERGEN
• Encase mattresses, pillows, and quilts in impermeable covers.
• Wash all bedding in the hot cycle (> 130° F) weekly.
• Replace carpets with tile, linoleum, or wood flooring.
• Minimize upholstered furniture/replace with leather furniture.
• Keep dust-accumulating objects in closed cupboards.
• Use a vacuum cleaner with an integral high efficiency particulate air (HEPA) filter and double-thickness bags.
• Replace curtains with blinds or easily washable (hot cycle) curtains.
• Hot wash or freeze soft toys.
Note. From National Heart, Lung, and Blood Institute/World Health Organization. (2003). *Global Initiative for Asthma: Global strategies for asthma management and prevention.* (NIH Publication No. 02-3659). Retrieved September 12, 2002, from http://www.ginasthma.com

Several measures families may use for control of mites are not effective. Mitocides have become widely advertised, and although they remove the mite allergen, they do not remove the mite itself, so they are not recommended (NHLBI, 1997). Air filtration units are not effective in reducing mite exposure because mites are aerodynamic (NHLBI/WHO, 2003).

Animal Allergens

All warm-blooded pets produce dander, urine, feces, and saliva that can cause allergic reactions. Cat allergen is a particularly potent airway-sensitizing agent. Cat allergen easily becomes airborne and sensitized persons become symptomatic almost immediately after exposure. Cat allergen can be found in concentrations high enough to produce symptoms even in places where no cat is present. Cat owners carry cat allergen on their clothes and transport it to public places such as schools, hospitals, and restaurants.

Dog and domestic bird allergens may act as triggers but are not as potent as cat allergen (HPDP/IOM, 2004). The best animal allergen avoidance strategy is to remove the pet from the home; however, families must understand that it may take months to remove the reservoir. If the family is unwilling to remove the pet, they should be advised to keep the pet out of the bedroom, close the bedroom door, remove upholstered furniture and carpet, or isolate the pet from the affected individual. Pets can be washed twice weekly, but this is only partially effective.

See Table 6-2 for measures to reduce exposure to animal allergens.

Cockroaches

Cockroaches are a problem, especially in inner cities. Most control measures are only partially effective, especially in multi-unit dwellings. However, all cracks should be sealed, dampness should be controlled, and food and garbage should be removed. Baits are recommended over insecticide sprays because sprays are inhaled and are irritating to the airway.

TABLE 6-2: MEASURES FOR REDUCING EXPOSURE TO ANIMAL ALLERGEN

- Keep the pet out of the main living areas and bedroom.
- Install high efficiency particulate air (HEPA) air cleaners in the main living areas and bedroom.
- Have the pet washed twice per week. (Some studies report this to be ineffective.)
- Thoroughly clean upholstered furniture/replace with leather furniture.
- Replace carpets with tile, linoleum, or wood flooring.
- Use a vacuum cleaner with integral HEPA filter and double-thickness bags.

Note. From National Heart, Lung and Blood Institute/World Health Organization. (2003). *Global Initiative for Asthma: Global strategies for asthma management and prevention.* (NIH Publication No. 02-3659). Retrieved September 12, 2002, from http://www.ginasthma.com

Fungi

Visible indoor fungi are called mold or mildew. Fungi reproduce by producing spores, which are regularly found in indoor air and on surfaces. Airborne spores are inhaled and act as allergens. Mold is usually accompanied by bacterial growth and has inflammatory effects. Although no indoor space is free of fungi, it is more likely to be found in homes older than 10 years, or homes with recent water damage and inadequate heating and ventilation (Zock, Jarvis, Luczynska, Sunyer, & Burney, 2002). House plant soil is also a source of indoor mold.

Moisture is the prime factor that controls growth of indoor mold. Mold can be limited by controlling dampness, maintaining indoor humidity below 50%, controlling condensation, repairing leaks, and replacing wet materials as soon as possible. Air conditioners and dehumidifiers are helpful because they reduce humidity and filter large fungal spores. Central heating and venting ovens seem to be protective against mold growth (Zock et al., 2002).

There is currently great interest in studying the effect of indoor dampness on respiratory illnesses. This is a relatively new field of investigation and definitive guidelines are not available to date. However, from studies conducted thus far, there is evidence to suggest that dampness and high indoor humidity are associated with the development of new onset asthma. Unfortunately, acceptable mold levels have not been identified and it is not clear what factors associated with damp environments (e.g., dust mites, cockroaches, mold, or bacteria), are responsible. There is also no current standard to assess the need for remediation and data on the effectiveness of remediation are lacking (HDPD, IOM, 2004).

Smoking

Smoke contains more than 4,500 contaminants and compounds and is the most important airway irritant. It is a major precipitator of asthma symptoms and increased medication use in children and adults. Smoke increases asthma severity and worsens lung function (Mannino, Homa, & Redd, 2002) and results in poor response to treatment and resistance to oral corticosteroids (Chaudhuri, et al., 2003).

Side stream, or second hand, smoke burns hotter and is more toxic than smoke inhaled by the user. Side stream smoke is particularly irritating to the respiratory tract. Passive maternal smoke is a risk factor for the development of new onset asthma in young children, and it intensifies symptoms and delays recovery from attacks in older children.

Avoidance strategies are to stop smoking. Environmental home visits and studies that measure urinary cotinine (a biologic marker for nicotine) indicate that denial of smoking is high among patients and families. The questioning technique used in these studies may affect reliability of data. Individuals should be asked, "Who smokes in the home?" rather than, "Does anyone smoke at home?" Also, families should be asked about smoking in the car. Parents who are unable to stop smoking should be told not to smoke in the house. This is only partially effective because smoke is carried inside on clothes. Smokers should be referred to smoking cessation programs. The American Lung Association has a free on-line "Freedom from Smoking®" program available at www.lungusa.org.

Indoor Pollutants

Indoor pollutants, such as carbon monoxide, carbon dioxide, and nitrogen oxide, are produced by cooking with natural gas, liquid propane, wood, or coal burning stoves; heating with gas, coal, or wood; and use of fireplaces. Building and furnishing materials such as foam insulation, glues, fireboard, pressed board, plywood, particleboard, carpet backing, paint, and products containing formaldehyde also produce indoor pollutants. As discussed earlier, improved sealing and insulation of modern buildings prevents ventilation and diffusion of these products to the outdoors.

Strategies to reduce levels of indoor pollutants include venting furnaces and gas appliances to the outside, avoiding wood smoke, adequately ventilating the home, and avoiding all household sprays including hair spray and furniture polishes (NHLBI/WHO, 2003). Mobile homes are constructed with many products that emit indoor pollutants, especially formaldehyde from particleboard. If possible, patients should move to a different type of dwelling or keep the mobile home well ventilated.

OUTDOOR TRIGGERS

Pollen and Molds

Pollen and molds are impossible to avoid completely. Outdoor mold is found in moist areas, such as in wet leaves and woodpiles. Standing moisture, wet leaves, and woodpiles should be removed from around the home.

Common sources of pollen are trees, grasses, and weeds. Concentration of pollen varies with weather conditions, location, and season. In general, tree pollen predominates in early spring; grass in late spring and summer; and weed in summer and fall. Avoidance strategies include remaining indoors when pollen counts are high and keeping windows closed, especially during the middle of the day and afternoon when pollen counts are highest.

Air Pollution

There is a significant association of pollution with asthma exacerbations and allergic responses. Air pollution has two sources: industrial and photochemical smog. Manufacturing industries emit sulfur dioxide, a major component of industrial smog. Traffic produces exhaust composed of ozone and nitrogen oxides and is an example of photochemical smog. The amount of smog in the air is affected by weather and geographic conditions. For example, ozone levels rise dramatically in hot weather.

Air pollution has been difficult to study because of shifting wind conditions and methodological problems. Improved measurement methodologies have recently been developed, and there is currently great interest in studying the effects of air pollution on respiratory health. Clinical experience seems to indicate that patients who live close to sources of industrial pollution suffer more severe asthma. Epidemiologists are designing studies to verify this impression by geographic mapping areas of high asthma incidence. Hopefully these studies will provide data for improved air quality standards.

Weather Changes

Sudden changes in the weather are problematic for many patients with asthma. The shift from warm to cold weather is especially difficult. In fact, the late fall and winter months are often referred to as "asthma season." Emergency room and urgent care visits are highest at these times of year. Patients who react to weather changes should be taught to monitor peak flow and start or increase their controller medication several weeks before the anticipated weather change.

Other Factors

Food rarely acts as an asthma trigger except in young children. Food avoidance is not recommended before a food challenge is carried out. Sulfites, preservatives in processed foods (such as potatoes, shrimp, dried fruits, beer, and wine) can cause severe asthma and even death. Fortunately; sulfites are no longer widely used.

Viruses, especially respiratory synctial, rhinovirus, and influenza viruses cause inflammation and damage to the airway epithelium and exacerbation of asthma. A clear association has been found between severe respiratory viral infections in early life and the development of asthma. Patients should be taught to avoid persons with colds, get sufficient sleep and nourishment, and receive the annual influenza vaccine.

Extreme emotional expression, such as laughing, crying, and panic, causes hyperventilation and hypocapnia. These events lead to airway narrowing.

Panic is often a natural response to acute asthma attacks. Relaxation techniques should be taught to persons who tend to panic. (See chapter 15 for a discussion of relaxation.)

Drugs such as aspirin, nonsteroidal anti-inflammatory agents, and beta-blockers can act as asthma triggers. These drugs are primarily used by adults and are discussed further in chapter 9. Heroin insufflation (snorting) is a common cause of intensive care admission in inner-city patients with life threatening asthma. Patients admitted to an intensive care unit should be asked about heroin use and referred to a rehabilitation program (Krantz, Hershow, Prachand, Hayden, Franklin, & Hryhorczuk, 2003).

IMMUNOTHERAPY

Immunotherapy can be considered for individuals sensitive to a particular allergen when there is a clear relationship between symptoms and unavoidable exposure to allergens. Generally, immunotherapy is recommended for those who suffer symptoms year round or a major part of the year and for individuals whose asthma is difficult to control with medication. Immunotherapy is carried out in a physician's office with trained personnel. Equipment is readily available to treat a life-threatening reaction. Bronchoconstriction is a common response to immunotherapy in patients with asthma. Immunotherapy is a long-term therapy, occurring over 3 to 5 years, but it does lead to a reduction in symptoms.

THE NURSE'S ROLE IN TRIGGER MANAGEMENT EDUCATION

Many people with asthma have difficulty identifying their triggers. The nurse can assist the patient by exploring with them "what happens" when they come in contact with a potential trigger. For instance, does playing with a cat produce an itchy nose, sneezing, and coughing? Does attending a barbeque result in a tight chest? What happens to the patient's breathing after a sudden change in the weather? These questions may be difficult for the patient to answer initially. Even though these questions may not yield immediate information, they are important to ask because they serve to increase symptom awareness during future contacts with triggers. Suggested trigger assessment questions are listed in Table 6-3.

Another strategy to identify triggers is to conduct an environmental assessment of the home. A home assessment is conducted by systematically walking through the grounds and each room of the house and checking for odors, signs of moisture, mold, dust, presence of pets or roaches, and adequate ventilation systems and control measures. A number of home assessment tools are available, but some are complicated to use or expensive. The Finger Lakes Environmental Home Assessment (Table 6-4) is a concise, one-page tool that targets

TABLE 6-3: ASSESSMENT QUESTIONS FOR ENVIRONMENTAL TRIGGERS

Inhalant Allergens

Does the patient have symptoms year round?

- Does the patient keep pets indoors? What type?
- Does the patient have moisture or dampness in any room of the house?
- Is mold visible in any part of the house?
- Have cockroaches been seen in the house in the last month?
- (Assume exposure to dust mites unless the patient lives in an arid climate.)

Do symptoms get worse at certain times of the year?

- Early spring (trees)
- Late spring (grasses)
- Late summer to autumn (weeds)
- Summer and autumn (fungi)

Tobacco Smoke

- Does the patient smoke?
- Does anyone smoke at home or work?
- Does anyone smoke at the child's daycare?

Indoor/Outdoor Pollutants and Irritants

- Is a wood-burning stove or fireplace used in the home?
- Are there unvented stoves or heaters in the home?
- Does the patient have contact with other smells or fumes from perfumes, cleaning agents, or sprays?

Rhinitis

Does the patient have constant or seasonal nasal congestion and/or postnasal drip?

Note. Adapted from National Asthma Education and Prevention Program. (1997). Expert panel report 2. *Guidelines for the diagnosis and management of asthma.* (NIH Publication No. 97-4051). Bethesda, MD: National Institutes of Health, National Heart, Lung, and Blood Institute. Available online at www.nhlbi.nih.gov/guidelines/asthma/index.pdf

key asthma triggers. This tool can be easily downloaded from the Web site of the Regional Community Asthma Network of The Finger Lakes. Some practices request the local health department

TABLE 6-4: ENVIRONMENTAL HOME ASSESSMENT

ENVIRONMENTAL HOME ASSESSMENT

Name_____ DOB _____ Parent/Guardian: _____

Address _____Apt #_____ Zip code _____

List numbers where family can be contacted _____

Referral Source _____ Reason for Referral _____

School Name & Contact _____Phone_____Fax_____

Dwelling Characteristics
House   Duplex   Mobile Home   Other_____
Apartment – Location   Rented   Owned

General Housekeeping: **Cleanliness:**   Very Clean   Clean   Other
Cleaning Frequency: Daily   Every Other Day   Weekly
   Other Cleaning Materials Used: _____
Dust Level: None noted   Some   Moderate   Substantial
Floors damp mopped: Daily   Weekly   Monthly   Other _____
Vacuuming frequency: Daily   Weekly   Monthly   Other _____
Type of vacuum: _____ Age of Vacuum: _____ Freq. of bag change _____ Hepa filter
Clutter/Debris/Garbage/Food: None   Some   Moderate   Substantial
Laundry: Laundromat   Home-   Hot Water Cycle used on Bedding   Gas dryer   Electric dryer

---

Floors, Furniture & Window Coverings:
Carpeting: Rooms: _____   Wet carpets   Deodorizers used on carpet
Hardwood Floors/Tile/Vinyl: Rooms: _____
Throw Rugs: Rooms: _____   Dirt Floors: Rooms: _____
Upholstered Furniture: Rooms _____
Curtains   Blinds   Drapes   Shades   Blankets   Other _____
Evidence of chipping/ pealing paint

Triggers:
Smoker in the Home
   Smokes in the House   One room of House   Car
Cats _____   Dogs _____   Birds _____
Cockroaches   Rodents
Candles/Incense   Aerosol Sprays   Room Deodorizer
Interior Plants: Type if known _____
Quilt   Curtains: Type_____
Mold or Mildew Noted: List where _____
Evidence of wet/ moist Carpets   Standing Water: List Where _____
Roof Leaks   Plumbing Leaks   Stained Ceilings   Stained Walls   Other _____

Client's Bedroom: _____
First floor   Second floor   Basement
Mattress on Bed   On Floor   Sofa
Dust Proof Encasings Present
Pillow   Feather   Foam
Bedding   Sheets   Blankets   Comforter
Stuffed Animals

Heating, Ventilation, Cooling and Air Conditioning:
Heating System: Gas Furnace   Oil Furnace   Electric Furnace   Coal/ Wood Stove   Floor Radiant   Electric
Baseboard   Fire Place   Kerosene Space Heaters   Kitchen Range   other:_____
Distribution System: Forced Air   Hot Water/Steam Radiator   Hot Water Baseboard   Room Fans
   Furnace Filter present: Type: Fiberglass   Hi-Efficiency   Electronic   Hepa
   Filter Changed or Cleaned: Monthly   Quarterly   Semi-annual   Annual   Other:_____
Cooking: Gas   Elec.   **Water Heater:**   Gas   Elec.   **Air Conditioning:**   Central   Window
   Dehumidifier in Basement   Humidifier Used   Vaporizer Used   Portable Air Cleaners   Bathroom
Exhaust Fan   Kitchen Range Exhaust Fan   Dryer Vented Outside

---

Completed By: Name/Title: _____ Date: _____
Agency: _____ Phone: _____

Developed by the Regional Community Asthma Network of the Finger Lakes (RCAN)
Produced with funding from the New York State Department of Health. Bureau of Child and Adolescent Health 10/04

Note. From Finger Lakes Environmental Home Assessment. Printed with permission of Regional Community Asthma Network of the Finger Lakes: www.rcanasthma.net

to assign a nurse to make a home visit. Another alternative is to request support from schools of nursing through their community health courses. Finally, depending on their capabilities and motivation, the family members may be able to complete the assessment.

Nurses should teach patients that asthma symptoms cannot be adequately controlled by medication alone. Patients must understand the importance of trigger avoidance. A recent survey of parents of children with asthma regarding use of trigger control methods found that most parents made an effort to control triggers, but only half of the measures parents used were recommended by the National Asthma Education and Prevention Program Guidelines (Cabana et al., 2004). At least half of the measures used were not effective for the child's specific trigger. For example, many parents purchased air filters even though filtering did not eliminate the trigger. Many purchased humidifiers, a strategy that is not recommended. Few families with a smoker attempted to reduce the smoke. However, frequency of office visits and asthma education resulted in action to control triggers.

The nurse should identify recommended strategies that are appropriate to the patient's unique trigger profile. Assist the family in identifying and eliminating triggers. Focus on the bedroom. Recommend strategies that are the least expensive as an initial strategy, such as damp mopping and washing bedding on a weekly basis. Costly alternatives, such as purchase of allergy covers for the bedding, can be recommended if initial strategies fail to reduce symptoms.

Finally, the nurse should be sensitive to difficulties encountered by patients and families when attempting to implement trigger control strategies. Environmental control strategies are difficult to implement for various reasons, such as emotional attachment to pets, lack of authority to remove carpets or clean air ducts in rental units, installation expense for alternative flooring, or relocating from a mobile home. Families do state their appreciation when nurses provide trigger education with an empathetic approach.

SUMMARY

Trigger avoidance is the most important asthma control measure. Triggers are classified as irritants or allergens because they evoke different asthma responses. Inhaled allergens are the most important triggers, but they evoke a response only in those who are sensitized to a particular allergen. Sensitivity is determined by the individual's genetic profile.

Triggers are further classified as indoor or outdoor. Most control measures focus on control of indoor triggers, especially in the bedroom. Common triggers and control strategies were reviewed. The nurse has an important role in assisting patients and families in identifying and avoiding triggers.

CASE STUDY

Jeremy, age 10, has mild persistent asthma. His triggers are cold weather, smoke, upper respiratory tract infections (URIs) and dust. After the weather suddenly became cold and wet, Jeremy experienced an acute asthma attack that resulted in an emergency room (ER) visit. Findings from a home visit revealed smoke damage to half of the house from a recent fire. The family moved into the home because the rent was reduced due to fire damage. Other findings included cigarette smoking by the mother limited to her own bedroom, clutter in Jeremy's bedroom, expired canisters of rescue medication, and a resolving URI for Jeremy. The mother was stressed financially and emotionally and refused to discuss smoking cessation. When Jeremy experiences difficulty breathing, she lets him sleep in her room.

Answer the following study questions, writing your responses on a separate sheet of paper. Compare your responses with the answers located at the end of the chapter.

1. Could this ER visit have been prevented?

2. Considering the mother's stress and limited resources, describe a trigger control plan that Jeremy could reasonably follow.

3. What is the significance of the expired rescue inhalers?

4. What is the significance of the burned house?

Answers to Case Study

1. Most ER visits are preventable. A combination of recognition of early warning signs, trigger control, and prompt pharmacologic treatment results in adequate home management in most cases.

2. The nurse should stress trigger control measures that Jeremy can manage. He can control the bedroom clutter, recognize early warning signs, and notify an adult (including the school nurse) when he experiences warning signs. Jeremy should also avoid sleeping in the mother's room because it contains smoke. Ideally, the mother should stop smoking—or at least smoke outside the house, but she may not be willing to do this. Jeremy can also be taught to try to avoid people with colds and to practice frequent hand washing.

3. Jeremy had no rescue medication available. The nurse should stress to the mother the importance of keeping medication current. This may be an indication that she cannot afford medication and may not purchase controller medication. She may need help with resources to obtain medication. She will most likely not have the money to invest in costly trigger control strategies. Economical measures should be stressed.

4. Indoor air pollutants may be emitted from the burned part of the house. Certainly the home is substandard. As an advocate, the nurse should assist the family in identifying resources to help locate adequate housing.

EXAM QUESTIONS

CHAPTER 6
Questions 31-36

31. Response to asthma triggers is influenced genetically because

    a. a single asthma gene determines an individual's response to triggers.

    b. persons with the asthma gene have identical responses to allergens.

    c. multiple genes determine an individual's response to allergens.

    d. genes determine an individual's response to airway irritants.

32. Irritants differ from allergens in that irritants cause

    a. bronchoconstriction.

    b. severe asthma symptoms.

    c. airway inflammation.

    d. permanent airway damage.

33. A common asthma allergen is

    a. ozone.

    b. cold air.

    c. food.

    d. mold.

34. The most important location for trigger control is

    a. the child's school.

    b. highly industrialized areas

    c. the bedroom.

    d. damp areas around the outside of the home.

35. Sandy is allergic to dust mites and mold. A control strategy that is effective for both triggers is

    a. the use of aerosolized cleaning sprays.

    b. central heating.

    c. damp mopping.

    d. keeping humidity below 50%.

36. Trigger education is likely to be most effective when the nurse offers the family

    a. instructions to remove carpets.

    b. recommendations to purchase filtering equipment.

    c. sensitivity that these are difficult measures to implement.

    d. strategies to implement regardless of the costs.

REFERENCES

Board on Health Promotion and Disease Prevention, Institute of Medicine. (2004). *Damp indoor spaces and health.* [Electronic version] Washington, DC: The National Academies Press. Retrieved November 7, 2004, from, http://books.nap.edu

Cabana, M., Slish, K., Lewis, T., Brown, R., Bin N., Xihong L., & Clark, N. (2004). Parental management of asthma triggers within a child's environment. *Journal of Allergy and Clinical Immunology, 114,* 352-357.

Chaudhuri, R., Livingston, E., McMahon, A., Thompson, L., Borland, W., & Thompson, N. (2003). Cigarette smoking impairs the therapeutic response to oral corticosteroids in chronic asthma. *American Journal of Respiratory and Critical Care Medicine, 168,* 1308-1311.

Krantz, A., Hershow, R., Prachand, N., Hayden, D., Franklin, C., & Hryhorczuk, D. (2003). Heroin insufflation as a trigger for patients with life-threatening asthma. *Chest, 123*(2), 510-517.

Langley, S., Goldthorpe, S., Craven, M., Morris, J., Woodcock, A., & Custovic, A. (2003). Exposure and sensitization to indoor allergens: Association with lung function, bronchial reactivity, and exhaled nitric oxide measures in asthma. *Journal of Allergy and Clinical Immunology, 112*(2), 362-368.

Mannino, D., Homa, D., & Redd, S. (2002). Involuntary smoking and asthma severity in children: Data from the third national health and nutrition examination survey. *Chest, 122*(2), 409-415.

National Asthma Education and Prevention Program. (1997). Expert panel report 2. *Guidelines for the diagnosis and management of asthma.* (NIH Publication No. 97-4051). Bethesda, MD: National Institutes of Health, National Heart, Lung, and Blood Institute. Available online at www.nhlbi.nih.gov/guidelines/asthma/index.pdf

National Heart, Lung, and Blood Institute/World Health Organization. (2003). *Global Initiative for asthma: Global strategies for asthma management and prevention.* (NIH Publication No. 02-3659.) Retrieved September 12, 2002, from http://www.ginasthma.com

Zock, JP., Jarvis, D., Luczynska, C., Sunyer, J. & Burney, P. (2002). Housing characteristics, reported mold exposure, and asthma in the European community respiratory health survey. *Journal of Allergy and Clinical Immunology, 110,* 285-292.

CHAPTER 7

CARE OF THE CHILD WITH ASTHMA

CHAPTER OBJECTIVE

Upon completion of this chapter, the reader will be able to recognize how the child's stage of development impacts (or influences) asthma management.

LEARNING OBJECTIVES

After studying this chapter, the reader will be able to

1. recognize the natural history of asthma.

2. identify three risk factors for the development of asthma in children.

3. recognize two difficult issues concerning the diagnosis of asthma in infants and young children.

4. recognize appropriate asthma monitoring and management strategies for the child according to stage of development.

5. state the impact of childhood asthma on the family.

6. provide patient education from a developmental perspective.

OVERVIEW

General principles of asthma diagnosis, monitoring, pharmacotherapy, and environmental control were discussed in previous chapters. This chapter and the following two chapters discuss the application of asthma management at different points along the lifespan—childhood, pregnancy, and adulthood. This chapter focuses on childhood from infancy through adolescence. Throughout this chapter, infants refers to newborns to age 1 year, preschool refers to children ages 1 to 6, school age ranges from age 6 to puberty and adolescence ranges from puberty to age 18.

The basic pathology of asthma is the same in children as in adults, but there are important differences in anatomy, physiology, and drug metabolism, as well as developmental and psychosocial characteristics that warrant an examination of asthma from a pediatric perspective. A discussion of natural history sets the stage for comprehending presentation of asthma at different ages. Variations in care are discussed through a developmental and family perspective. It is essential for the nurse to apply developmental and family concepts in the care of children with asthma and their families.

NATURAL HISTORY OF ASTHMA

Wheezing is common in infants and preschoolers and can be caused by many different conditions. Because many infants who experience a wheeze do not develop asthma, it is thought that small lungs may be responsible for infant wheezing. Those children who continue to wheeze have atopy (the genetic predisposition to develop IgE in response to environmental triggers), allergy, and allergic rhinitis (National Heart, Lung, and Blood Institute/World Health Organization [NHLBI/WHO], 2003). Appearance of asthma symptoms before age 3 is associated with significant decline in lung function by late school age. There is current interest in targeting preventive therapy to children younger than age 3 to prevent irreversible lung changes, but it has not been possible to identify those children with wheeze who will develop asthma.

Because of the clinical variability seen in childhood wheezing and the need to identify therapeutic targets, attempts have been made to classify patterns of wheezing. Three patterns of wheezing have been identified, some of which progress to asthma: transient early wheezing, nonatopic wheezing, and atopic wheezing/asthma (Martinez, 2002). Transient early wheezing resolves by age 3 and is not associated with family history of asthma or allergy. Children at risk for transient early wheezing are premature infants, children in day care, children with exposure to siblings, and children exposed to maternal smoking during pregnancy or in the first few years of life.

Many school children have a history of nonatopic wheezing sometime in the first few years of life. The most common cause is viral infection, usually respiratory syncytial virus (RSV). RSV associated wheezing resolves in most children by age 13 and is not associated with allergic sensitization.

Approximately half of all children with persistent or atopic asthma develop symptoms before age 3 and 80% develop symptoms by age 8. Early allergic sensitization is a risk factor for persistent asthma. Onset of symptoms before age 3 is associated with increased asthma severity and decreased pulmonary function.

By age 8, a proportion of children develop moderate to severe persistent asthma, whereas some continue with mild intermittent asthma. Clinical symptoms of asthma disappear in 30% to 50% of children at puberty—especially in males. However, two thirds of adults experience a recurrence of symptoms. Even when asthma has clinically disappeared, lung function frequently remains altered and hyperresponsiveness and cough persist (NHLBI/WHO, 2003). It is thought that ongoing inflammation is the cause of the reappearance of asthma. This thinking is based on the observation that children who have asthma symptoms for more than 1 year have increased smooth muscle tone, hyperresponsiveness, inflammatory cells and airway wall thickening (van den Toorn, Overbeek, Prins, Hoogsteden, & Jongste, 2003). The important point here is that asthma should never be neglected in the hopes that the child will outgrow it.

Controversy exists over the use of inhaled corticosteroids (ICSs) in relation to the natural history of asthma. Because many postpubescent adolescents experience a remission of symptoms with a later reappearance as adults, it is being questioned whether ICSs should be continued in the absence of symptoms (van den Toorn et al., 2003). It has also been observed that by the time childhood asthma is diagnosed, usually around age 5, the inflammatory process and airway remodeling is well underway. It is known that ICSs cannot reverse remodeling once it is present; however, the possibility that very early ICS therapy may have a role in preventing remodeling is being explored (Cohn, Elias, & Chupp, 2004).

RISK FACTORS FOR THE DEVELOPMENT OF ASTHMA IN THE CHILD

Genetics

Genetics influence the tendency to develop atopy and airway hyperresponsiveness. Atopy runs in families. When atopy is present, it is one of the strongest predictors of asthma. Commonly, parents provide the healthcare provider with a history of allergic rhinitis, atopic dermatitis, or asthma in one or both parents. The timing of allergic sensitization in the child and the development of asthma is age dependent. Most children who become sensitized to allergens in the first 3 years of life develop asthma, but sensitization to allergens after ages 8 to 10 carries less risk (NHLBI/WHO, 2003).

Gender

For children younger than age 10, risk of asthma is higher in boys than in girls. It is thought that boys have narrower airways, increased airway tone, and possibly higher serum IgE levels. This gender difference in asthma rates disappears after age 10, when the diameter and length ratio of the airway is the same in boys and girls. This is also the age when boys experience growth in the size of the thoracic cage. After puberty, asthma is more common in girls (NHLIB/WHO, 2003).

Viral Illness

Among preschoolers the most common cause of asthma symptoms is viral illness. Two symptom patterns have been identified in children who wheeze with upper respiratory illnesses (URIs) (National Asthma Education and Prevention Program Update [NAEPP], 2003). Children either have a remission of wheezing or progress to wheezing throughout childhood. Risk factors that predict continuation of wheezing include three episodes of wheezing throughout the previous year and either a physician diagnosis of atopic dermatitis (eczema) or a parental history of asthma. Alternatively, children who continue to wheeze into childhood may have two of the following three risk factors: high levels of eosinophils in the blood, wheezing in the absence of URIs, or a physician diagnosis of allergic rhinitis. Children with these risk factors have a 75% probability of asthma in the schoolage years.

Lack of Breast-feeding

Children younger than age 2 years who have ever been breast-fed may be actively protected or at least experience a delayed onset of asthma (Chulada, Arbes, Dunson, & Zeldin, 2003). Breast-feeding may also decrease the prevalence of asthma in children exposed to postnatal environmental tobacco smoke (ETS). However, prenatal ETS exposures are unaffected by breast-feeding.

It is hypothesized that the protective effect of breast-feeding may be attributed to a delay in allergic sensitization because the child is not exposed to foreign milk proteins. Breast milk also contains immunoglobulins that are essential for the development and maturation of the infant's immune system.

Environmental Tobacco Smoke

ETS is a lung irritant. Exposure to ETS leads to chronic inflammation of the airways and bronchoconstriction. Passive exposure is especially damaging because side stream smoke contains some toxins in higher quantities than mainstream smoke. Parental smoking is associated with higher prevalence rates of new onset asthma and more severe symptoms in children with the disease. In addition to more severe symptoms, children exposed to ETS have higher rates of emergency room visits and life-threatening asthma attacks (Committee on the Assessment of Asthma and Indoor Air, Institute of Medicine, 2000).

DIAGNOSIS IN INFANTS AND YOUNG CHILDREN

Diagnosis of asthma in infants and young children is challenging. The likelihood of an alternative diagnosis increases with younger age. As discussed above, wheezing is very common in infants and preschoolers. A wheeze is simply a sound produced by air passing through a narrow space. Airways of young children are narrow and are easily obstructed by mucus plugs associated with viral illnesses. Other conditions that produce narrowing of the airway include cystic fibrosis, foreign body, or immunodeficiency diseases, to name a few. Such narrowing leads to wheezing.

Asthma is commonly misdiagnosed as a form of bronchitis in young children. This is problematic because it results in mistreatment with antibiotics or cough medicines. Some physicians are reluctant to use the label "asthma" and use the term "reactive airway disease," or RAD, as an alternative diagnosis. This label is confusing and misleading. RAD is a distinct syndrome seen in adults that produces severe asthma-like symptoms after a one time exposure to an irritant. Healthcare providers are encouraged to use the word "asthma," even though certainty about development of persistent disease may be unclear.

The child with a viral-related wheeze should receive the diagnosis of asthma because the risk of overtreatment is balanced by the potential to shorten and reduce the intensity of wheezing episodes by effective use of asthma medications rather than with antibiotics (NHLBI/WHO, 2003). Furthermore, trust is built when parents are given accurate information. Breathing difficulty in young children produces anxiety but correct information helps parents deal with anxiety by facilitating the development of action plans and coping skills.

Diagnosis in young children is based on history, symptoms, the physical examination, and exclusion of other diagnoses. Exercise intolerance can be assessed by asking about wheezing or coughing when running, excitement, laughing, or crying. Young children are developmentally unable to perform objective tests of lung function, and many times the diagnosis is based on clinical judgment. Sometimes the child's response to a trial of asthma medication is necessary to establish the diagnosis.

School-age children are less challenging to diagnose because seasonal variation in symptom presentation becomes more evident and they are usually able to perform spirometry. However, a common pattern of symptom presentation in children is recurrent cough only, especially at night or with exercise—the so-called "cough variant asth-ma." It should be kept in mind that presence of a wheeze is not necessary for the diagnosis of asthma.

DEVELOPMENTALLY BASED ASTHMA CARE

Goals of Management

General goals of asthma management apply to children but some additional goals are needed. With asthma management, infants should feed, sleep, and grow normally. Although undisturbed sleep is important at all ages, it is especially important for school-age children because lack of sleep can affect academic performance. In addition, children should be able to engage fully in age appropriate activity, whether that means play or active involvement in sports.

Symptom Monitoring in Children

It is difficult to detect early warning signs in infants and preschoolers. To complicate detection difficulties, children this age rarely communicate the need for rescue medication. Parents of infants and preschoolers must be taught signs of respiratory distress. In addition to cough and wheeze, parents of infants and preschoolers must be taught to recognize other signs of respiratory distress, such as increased respiratory rate for the child's age, difficulty talking or lying down, trouble with feeding (in infants), softer or shorter cry, retracting, nasal flaring, agitation, and decreased responsiveness to the environment. The nurse should help parents identify early signs and intervene promptly. Retracting, difficulty speaking in phrases, and cyanosis are late signs. Breathlessness severe enough to interfere with feeding is an important sign of impending respiratory distress in infants.

Children who can blow out the candles on a birthday cake, usually 4- to 5-year-olds, are able to perform peak flow maneuvers. Parents need to supervise when and how children take peak flow measurements for reliability. School-age children want to be normal. They often ignore the early warning signs until symptoms interfere with activity. Education needs to be periodically reinforced to prompt the child to attend to early warning signs and tell an adult. Parents of school-age children sometimes express difficulty distinguishing asthma from nonasthma symptoms. They should be encouraged to use peak flow monitoring in these cases. Parents also tend to fail to recognize nocturnal cough as a symptom of poor asthma control (Meng & McConnell, 2002).

Adolescents commonly have the misperception that they have outgrown their asthma and thus may fail to identify symptoms. On the other hand, adolescents tend to use denial or minimizing as a coping strategy. These are maladaptive strategies and may lead to exacerbations severe enough to require hospitalization. It should be stressed that asthma never truly goes away.

Symptom recognition presents different challenges at every developmental stage. These difficulties provide a strong argument for the need for controller medication rather than as-needed rescue medication.

Application of Pharmacotherapy Principles in Children

Long-term studies in school-age children provide strong evidence for the efficacy of ICSs on health outcomes. To date, no studies have been conducted on children younger than age 5; therefore, data are extrapolated for this group. A potential side effect of chronic steroid therapy in children is delayed growth. In the past, media attention to this concern aroused anxiety about stunted growth in children with asthma. Since then, multiple studies have demonstrated that children treated with recommended dosages of corticosteroids achieve expected adult height (NAEPP, 2002). At the initiation of corticosteroid therapy, there is a slight (1 cm) delay in growth velocity, but catch up is achieved later. However, it must be noted that children with

untreated asthma also experience delayed growth. The small risk of delayed growth from ICS therapy is well balanced by its effectiveness. At recommended dosages no other clinically significant side effects are associated with ICS therapy and no other class of medication is as effective in controlling asthma as the corticosteroids.

Recommendations for the use of asthma medications are summarized in Tables 7-1 and 7-2. Table 7-1 lists medications with age-related recommendations. Table 7-2 lists therapy recommendations based on disease severity in young children (see Tables 5-1 through 5-3 for recommendations in children older than age 5).

Because of the diagnostic dilemmas in young children discussed above, it is sometimes difficult to determine whether controller therapy is needed. Recommendations for use of ICSs in young children are based on studies of wheezing in early childhood. Long-term controller therapy with ICSs should be considered in infants and young children with asthma risk factors who experience more than three episodes of wheezing in 1 year that last more than 1 day and affect sleep. Daily controller therapy is also recommended for young children who consistently require rescue medication more than two times per week and for young children who experience severe exacerbations that occur less than 6 weeks apart (NAEPP, 2003). When asthma control is sustained and no symptoms are present for 2 to 4 weeks, a gradual decrease in the corticosteroid dose can be considered.

Side effects of ICSs, although small, are sometimes evident in the medium-dose range. For this reason, the addition of long-acting bronchodilators (LAB) to low-dose ICS therapy is preferred for children with moderate or severe persistent asthma. There are no data on the use of combination therapy with ICS and LABs in children younger than age 4, but studies do show that medium-dose ICS therapy is effective for moderate to severe persistent asthma in young children.

TABLE 7-1: AGE-RELATED MEDICATION RECOMMENDATIONS FOR THE TREATMENT OF ASTHMA IN CHILDREN

Medication	Recommendation
Nonsteroidals:	
Cromolyn sodium Nedocromil	No longer recommended as initial treatment; insufficient data on benefits; alternative treatment for mild persistent asthma and prior to exercise
Controller Medications:	
Budesonide	Nebulized solution approved by the Food and Drug Administration (FDA) for children older than age 1 year
Fluticasone dry-powdered inhaler	FDA approved for ages 4 years and above
Salmeterol dry-powdered inhaler	FDA approved for ages 4 years and above
Montelukast 4 mg chewable 5 mg	FDA approved for ages 2 to 5 years For ages 6 to 14 years
Fluticasone/Salmeterol dry-powdered inhaler	FDA approved for ages 4 years and above
Theophylline sustained-release	Not recommended as long-term control in young children with mild persistent asthma; can be considered as adjunct therapy in moderate to severe asthma if cost is a factor, but serum levels must be carefully monitored.
Leukotriene Modifiers:	Alternative, not preferred treatment for mild persistent asthma
Montelukast	Available for children older than age 2 years
Zafirlukast	Available for children older than age 7 years
Zileuton	Available for children older than age 12 years

Note. Adapted from National Asthma Education and Prevention Program. (2003). Expert Panel Report. *Guidelines for the diagnosis and management of asthma: Update on selected topics 2002.* (NIH Publication No. 02-5074). Bethesda, MD: National Institutes of Health, National Heart, Lung and Blood Institute. Available online at http://www.nhlbi.nih.gov/guidelines/asthma/index.htm

Asthma exacerbations triggered by viral illness can be severe. Regardless of presence or absence of risk factors for persistent asthma, young children with a viral-associated, severe exacerbation should be treated with systemic corticosteroids. Children who have no symptoms between viral illnesses do not need maintenance ICS therapy because corticosteroids do not prevent exacerbations caused by viruses (Weinberger, 2003).

The leukotriene modifier, montelukast, is approved for the treatment of asthma in children ages 2 and older and has the advantage of once daily dosing by mouth. The pediatric dose is 4 or 5 mg once daily. This dose is pharmacokinetically comparable to the 10-mg dose used in adults. Food does not affect bioavailability of montelukast. Montelukast is more effective than placebo but is not as effective as the corticosteroids (NHLBI/WHO, 2003).

A primary care provider can treat most children with asthma. However, if a child has a life-threatening event, fails to respond to therapy, or needs asthma education, the child should be referred to a specialist in allergy or pulmonary medicine.

Techniques of Medication Administration

It is not unusual to see treatment failures in children who are on optimal controller therapy. Faulty technique results in loss of medication delivery to

TABLE 7-2: A STEPWISE APPROACH FOR MANAGING INFANTS AND CHILDREN YOUNGER THAN AGE 5 YEARS WITH ACUTE OR CHRONIC ASTHMA

Severity Level	Symptoms/Day Symptoms/Night	Daily Medications
Step 4 Severe Persistent	continual daily frequent night	Preferred Treatment: High-dose inhaled corticosteroid (ICS) AND long-acting inhaled (beta$_2$-agonists, AND, if needed, corticosteroid tablets or syrup (2 mg/kg/day, generally not to exceed 60 mg/day)
Step 3 Moderate Persistent	daily > 1 night/week	Preferred Treatment: Low-dose ICS and long-acting bronchodilator (LAB) OR medium-dose ICS. Alternative Treatment: Low-dose ICS and leukotriene modifier or theophylline If needed (in patients with recurring severe exacerbations): Medium dose-ICS and LAB (preferred) OR medium-dose ICS and leukotriene modifier or theophylline
Step 2 Mild Persistent	> 2/week but < 1x/day > 2 nights/month	Preferred Treatment: Low dose ICS (with nebulizer and holding chamber with or without face mask or dry powder inhaler Alternative Treatment: Cromolyn (nebulizer preferred or metered-dose inhaler with holding chamber) OR leukotriene receptor antagonist
Step 1 Mild	< 2 days/week ≤ 2 nights/month	No daily medication needed

Note. Adapted from National Asthma Education and Prevention Program. (2003). Expert Panel Report. *Guidelines for the diagnosis and management of asthma: Update on selected topics 2002.* (NIH Publication No. 02-5074). Bethesda, MD: National Institutes of Health, National Heart, Lung and Blood Institute. Available online at http://www.nhlbi.nih.gov/guidelines/asthma/index.htm

the lungs. For instance, to correctly administer medication from a nebulizer, the facemask must fit tightly. Holding the facemask 1 cm away from the face results in a 50% loss of medication. Before the dose of medication is increased, technique of administration should be reviewed with the child and parents.

Choice of medication delivery device is based on the developmental ability of the child. Simplicity of operation is important for infants and young children because they are often uncooperative and they may be cared for by several different people throughout the day. Many parents prefer using nebulizers for young children, but this delivery system is not preferred for routine maintenance therapy. Nebulizers are bulky, time consuming, require cleaning, and give imprecise dosing unless

equipped with a dosimeter (NHLBI/WHO, 2003). Nebulizers are preferred during an acute attack because no cooperation is required from the child and accuracy of dosing is not critical at this time.

Metered-dose inhalers (MDIs) with spacers and facemasks are preferred for maintenance even in infants and preschoolers. Spacers with facemasks are available in infant and preschool sizes. Around ages 4 to 6 years, the child can be taught to use a spacer with mouthpiece. Parents often have success introducing a new device if they introduce it gradually and wean the child from the familiar device.

After age 6, the child may be given a dry powdered inhaler (DPI) if he has sufficient inspiratory force to generate medication delivery. Inspiratory force can be measured with the In-Check Dial.™

(See chapter 5 for a discussion of the In-Check dial™). Oral candidiasis may be seen in children on an ICS who are also receiving antibiotics. Correct inhaler technique, use of spacers, and rinsing and spitting after dosing reduce the risk of candidiasis.

Inhaler techniques tend to deteriorate over time. Correct technique should be assessed and reinforced at every healthcare visit.

IMPACT OF CHILDHOOD ASTHMA ON THE FAMILY

Childhood asthma affects the family in various ways. For example, breathlessness in a child is anxiety producing. Many parents of children with asthma, especially mothers, become hypervigilent. Anxiety is particularly notable in parents who have not coped with asthma themselves (Calam, Gregg, Simpson, Morris, Woodcock, & Custovia, 2003) and in parents of infants and young children. Another factor is that young children do not communicate the need for medication. Also, symptoms tend to occur at night, resulting in sleeplessness for the child and parents.

Parents' sense of confidence is a factor that can influence their assessment and management of the child (Svavarsdóttir & Rayens, 2003). The nurse should discuss the parents' perceptions of their ability to detect symptoms in their child, assess demands on the family, and support their management skills so that family members develop a belief in their ability to manage episodes of breathlessness. In addition, families should always have a telephone number to access a healthcare provider who is available around the clock to validate decision-making. Accessibility to a healthcare provider is especially important for newly diagnosed children because parents new to asthma management lack confidence in their decision-making skills.

Behavioral problems have been documented in children with asthma, particularly when onset of asthma occurs before age 6. The family is affected because parents may experience difficult interactions with the child out of fear that treatment disagreements will set off crying and breathing difficulties. They may retreat to avoid conflict (Calam, et al., 2003). The nurse should explore behavioral issues and teach the parents to stay calm and administer treatments with gentle authority.

Another issue is that parents assume or delegate asthma management tasks to the child inappropriately. Parents need education regarding age-appropriate involvement in care. The preschooler can be taught to label symptoms but it is not until age 6 or 7 that the child is ready to assume responsibility for care. At this age, the child can be taught to report symptoms and take medicines correctly (with reminders from the adult). By age 8, the child can request medication at the appropriate time, perform and record peak flow readings, and report early warning signs. The 9- to 10-year-old child can be expected to know the names of asthma medications and their correct use. The 11- to 12-year-old child is beginning to think abstractly and can assess his condition before and after treatments. Adolescents have the ability to manage all aspects of care. Parents should understand that regardless of the child's age, they have a role in care. Parents need to keep themselves informed regarding symptoms the child is experiencing, frequency of use of rescue and controller medication. Parents should also ensure that medication is on hand and schedule periodic clinic visits.

ASSISTING THE FAMILY IN COMMUNICATING WITH OTHER CARETAKERS

Children spend most of their day in school or day care. Parents of children with asthma sometimes have difficulty communicating the child's needs to the school. The nurse should ensure that the family has a simple, written personal action plan that summarizes specific actions to take if the child experiences symptoms at school. An emergency contact number needs to be included on the plan. The American Lung Association has an Asthma Individual Health Plan and a School Emergency Asthma Plan that can assist families communicating the child's asthma needs to the school. (See the resources listed at the end of the book for the American Lung Association's Web address.)

Schools contain many potential asthma triggers—chalk dust, strong smelling art or science materials, mold in showers and locker rooms, pets or plants in the classroom, and possible viral exposures. Parents should be instructed to provide the school with a list of the child's triggers and avoidance strategies. Rescue medication with a spacer should be available in the school. Depending on state law, students may be permitted to carry their own rescue medication. In such cases the child should be instructed to tell an adult when he needs to use rescue medication so that frequency of use can be monitored to assure that asthma control is maintained.

Some school nurses have noted that many children with asthma are not adhering to daily controller medication administration. Some schools have become proactive in administering controller medication at school. Students who received controller medication at school were noted to have more symptom free days and fewer absences (Halterman Szilagyi, Yoos, Conn, Kaczorowski, Holzhauer, et al., 2004). Nurses may be able to improve adherence by setting up a school administration program for those children who cannot adhere to home management.

SUMMARY

Natural history of asthma was discussed as a framework for presenting asthma at different stages of childhood. Risk factors for the development of asthma include genetic predisposition, gender, viral illness in the preschool years, lack of breast-feeding, and exposure to environmental tobacco smoke. The diagnosis of asthma is difficult to establish in infants and young children because young children commonly wheeze with many other conditions. Many infants who wheeze do not develop asthma. Nevertheless, treatment with an ICS is recommended for wheezing episodes to lessen the severity of the exacerbation.

Care of the child with asthma must be based on developmental principles. Symptom monitoring, pharmacology, and medication administration techniques were discussed from a developmental point of view. The impact of asthma on the family was also reviewed. Guidelines for age-appropriate child expectations and for communicating the asthma management plan to the school were also reviewed.

CASE STUDY

Jerry Brown, age 9, was seen in the clinic because his asthma symptoms worsened after the weather turned cold. His mother gave a history of three emergency room (ER) visits in the past 2 months. Jerry was previously seen 1 year ago but failed to keep appointments due to lack of insurance. His previous record indicated that he had mild persistent asthma and was well controlled on Flovent 44 mcg, 2 puffs twice per day. He has no medication on hand and stopped taking controller medication 11 months ago when the insurance expired.

Each recent ER visit documented reversal of symptoms with a single dose of nebulized albuterol. Mrs. Brown appeared anxious and confided that she was worried that Jerry's asthma had worsened. She added that several months ago her best friend died during an acute asthma attack. Spirometry indicated near normal lung function.

Answer the following study questions, writing your responses on a separate sheet of paper. Compare your responses with the answers located at the end of the chapter.

1. What are the indications that Jerry's asthma has worsened?

2. What impact has asthma had on Jerry's mother?

3. How would you instruct the mother to involve Jerry in care?

4. How can the nurse act as an advocate to ensure that Jerry has needed medication on hand?

Answers to Case Study

1. There are no indications that Jerry's asthma has worsened. The fact that he has no medication at home resulted in the emergency room visits. The treatment he received there could have been given at home. Jerry has a persistent form of asthma and needs daily controller medication for control of symptoms, especially during the cold weather season. If Jerry had been receiving controller medication, he most likely would not have needed to go to the ER. Spirometry confirms lack of progression of asthma.

2. Jerry's mother was anxious over his apparent worsening of symptoms. She failed to understand the preventive role of daily controller medication. Her anxiety was heightened by the death of her friend. Her coping skills were poor in that she did not call the clinic to communicate her problems obtaining medication.

3. Jerry should recognize and report early warning signs. He should know the names and correct uses of his asthma medications, take them on time, and monitor and record peak flow readings.

4. The nurse should confirm that the mother has a phone number for the healthcare provider. Many clinics have sample medications that can be used in emergency situations. The nurse may be able to facilitate application for Medicaid and recommend that the school nurse ensure that Jerry take his controller medication.

EXAM QUESTIONS

CHAPTER 7
Questions 37-42

37. Infants who wheeze are likely to develop asthma if they

    a. have two episodes of wheezing in the first 2 years of life.
    b. are exposed to viruses at day care.
    c. have parents who have allergy or asthma.
    d. have not received controller therapy early in life.

38. It is appropriate to label the diagnosis of the young child who presents with wheezing as

    a. asthma.
    b. bronchitis.
    c. RAD.
    d. pneumonia.

39. It is most difficult for parents to read early warning signs in

    a. infants.
    b. early school-age children.
    c. late school-age children.
    d. adolescents.

40. The most effective class of drugs for control of asthma in young children is

    a. nonsteroidal anti-inflammatory agents.
    b. leukotriene modifiers.
    c. long acting bronchodilators.
    d. ICSs

41. The preferred medication delivery method for infants is

    a. an MDI with spacer and face mask.
    b. a DPI.
    c. a nebulizer.
    d. oral syrups.

42. Children are developmentally ready to learn the names of their asthma medications at age

    a. 6 years old.
    b. 7 years old.
    c. 8 years old.
    d. 9 years old.

REFERENCES

Calam, R., Gregg, L., Simpson, B., Morris, J., Woodcock, A., & Custovic, A. (2003). Childhood asthma, behavior problems and family functioning. *Journal of Asthma and Clinical Immunology, 112*(3), 499-504.

Chulada, P., Arbes, S., Dunson, D., & Zeldin, D. (2003). Breastfeeding and the prevalence of asthma and wheeze in children: Analyses from the Third National Health and Nutrition Examination Survey. *Journal of Asthma and Clinical Immunology, 111*, 328-326.

Cohn, L., Elias, J., & Chupp, G. (2004). Asthma: Mechanisms of disease persistence and progression. *Annual Review of Immunology, 22*, 789-815.

Committee on the Assessment of Asthma and Indoor Air, Institute of Medicine. (2000). *Clearing the air: Asthma and indoor air exposures.* Washington, DC: National Academy Press.

Halterman, J., Szilagyi, P., Yoos, L., Conn, K., Kaczorowski, J., Holzhauer, R. et al. (2004). Benefits of a school-based asthma treatment program in the absence of second hand smoke exposure. *Archives of Pediatric Adolescent Medicine, 158*, 460-467.

Martinez, F. (2002). Development of wheezing disorders and asthma in preschool children. *Pediatrics, 109*(2), 362-367.

Meng, A. & McConnell, S. (2002). Decision-making in children with asthma and their parents. *Journal of the American Academy of Nurse Practitioners, 14*(8), 363-371.

National Asthma Education and Prevention Program. (2003). Expert Panel Report: *Guidelines for the diagnosis and management of asthma: Update on selected topics 2002.* (NIH Publication No. 02-5074). Bethesda, MD: National Institutes of Health, National Heart, Lung and Blood Institute. Available online at http://www.nhlbi.nih.gov/guidelines/asthma/index.html

National Heart, Lung, and Blood Institute/World Health Organization. (2003). *Global initiative for asthma: Global strategy for asthma management and prevention.* (NIH Publication No. 02-3659). Retrieved September 12, 2002, from http://www.ginasthma.com

Svavarsdóttir, E. & Rayens, M. (2003). American and Icelandic parents' perceptions of the health status of their young children with chronic asthma. *Journal of Nursing Scholarship, 35*(4), 351-358.

van den Toorn, L., Overbeek, S., Prins, J., Hoogsteden, H., & Jongste, J., (2003). Asthma remission: Does it exist? *Current Opinion in Pulmonary Medicine, 9*, 15-20.)

Weinberger, M. (2003). Clinical patterns and natural history of asthma. *Journal of Pediatrics, 142*(2S), s15-19.

CHAPTER 8

NURSING CARE OF THE WOMAN WITH ASTHMA DURING PREGNANCY

CHAPTER OBJECTIVE

Upon completion of this chapter, the reader will be able to identify how the course of asthma changes during pregnancy and how these changes impact asthma management.

LEARNING OBJECTIVES

After studying this chapter, the reader will be able to

1. recognize that asthma severity level may change during pregnancy.

2. state three goals of asthma management during pregnancy.

3. list five adverse outcomes to mother and child caused by poor asthma management.

4. identify five asthma medications that are safe during pregnancy.

5. recognize two nursing needs unique to antepartum and intrapartum asthma management.

6. identify five teaching needs of the childbearing woman with asthma.

OVERVIEW AND MANAGEMENT GOALS

Asthma is common in childbearing women, complicating as many as 7% of pregnancies (Schatz et al., 2004). Higher asthma rates are seen in younger women. This trend is predictive of an increase of asthma during pregnancy (Kwon, Belanger, & Bracken, 2004).

In approximately one third of women, asthma severity remains stable throughout pregnancy. Another third experience lessening of asthma severity, and the remaining third experience a worsening of symptoms (National Institutes of Health, National Heart, Lung, & Blood Institute [NIH/NHLBI], 1993). Women with more severe asthma tend to experience worsening of their asthma. However, the course of asthma during previous pregnancies can be predictive of asthma severity during the current pregnancy (Blaiss, 2004). With proper care, there is no increase in asthma-related mortality during pregnancy (NHLBI/World Health Organization [WHO], 2003).

Asthma management goals listed in Table 8-1 serve as a guide for safe and effective care during pregnancy. The most critical goal is to avoid fetal hypoxia because of its devastating effect on the fetus. Healthcare providers must provide close and careful monitoring of the mother with asthma and her fetus to achieve optimal management, to control symptoms, and to deliver a healthy infant (NHLBI/WHO, 2003). Guidelines for care during pregnancy have recently been revised and call for even more frequent monitoring than was recommended in the past (Blaiss, 2004).

TABLE 8-1: ASTHMA MANAGEMENT GOALS DURING PREGNANCY

1. Deliver a healthy infant.

2. Control asthma symptoms, including nocturnal symptoms.

3. Prevent acute exacerbations.

4. Prevent adverse medication reactions.

5. Maintain normal or near normal pulmonary functions.

6. Maintain normal activity levels including exercise.

(NIH/NHLBI, 1993)

MATERNAL PHYSIOLOGY AND POTENTIAL ADVERSE OUTCOMES

Normal physiologic changes during pregnancy influence fetal oxygenation. Total oxygen consumption, basal metabolic rate, cardiac output and blood volume increase during pregnancy. During an acute asthma exacerbation, maternal PO_2 may fall rapidly, causing a profound decrease in fetal oxygen saturation. In addition, maternal hyperventilation and hypocapnia may result in decreased blood flow to the uterus. Compensatory mechanisms will maintain blood pressure and oxygenation of vital maternal organs at the expense of uterine blood flow. Fetal distress can occur despite absence of maternal hypotension or hypoxia. Fetal status should be monitored continuously during treatment of asthma exacerbations (Gardner & Doyle, 2004).

Expansion of the rib cage and pressure from the uterus on the diaphragm in late pregnancy can result in shortness of breath or "dyspnea of pregnancy." This must be distinguished from the shortness of breath of asthma (Kwon, Belanger, & Bracken, 2004). Fortunately, common measures of pulmonary function do not change during pregnancy; therefore, altered test results indicate obstruction

and should be interpreted as asthma (NIH/NHLBI, 1993; Blaiss, 2004).

Increased progesterone production during pregnancy relaxes the lower esophageal sphincter and increases the risk of bronchospasm due to reflux. Maternal cell mediated immunosuppression may increase the risk of viral upper respiratory infections, which are the most common cause of asthma exacerbations during pregnancy. However, overall hormonal balance during pregnancy may have positive effects. Animal studies support the clinical observation that maternal hormones have a bronchodilating effect (Kwon, Belanger, & Bracken, 2004).

Asthma exacerbations tend to increase in the 24th to the 36th week of pregnancy but are rare in the last 4 weeks and during labor and delivery. These exacerbations should be treated aggressively because inadequate treatment results in adverse maternal and fetal outcomes (Dombrowski et al., 2004) such as preeclampsia, gestational hypertension, placenta previa, uterine hemorrhage, oligohydramnios, and increased risk of cesarean section (Blaiss, 2004). Risks to the infant include low birth weight, prematurity, and perinatal mortality (Blaiss, 2004).

PHARMACOTHERAPY

Risk Categories

Concern for fetal health and well-being heighten, especially when the mother has a chronic illness such as asthma. In the past, safety concerns have led some healthcare providers to stop asthma medications during pregnancy. This is not necessary and, in fact, is likely to lead to poor outcomes for mother and child. Good asthma control can be achieved with appropriate asthma medications at no additional risk to mother or infant. Controlled asthma results in the same fetal prognosis as in women without asthma. Therefore, "the use of asthma medications to achieve optimal asthma control is justified, even when safety has not been unequivocally proven" (NIH/NHLBI, 1993).

Fortunately, most drugs used to treat asthma fail to show increased risk to the fetus. Because few drug studies have been conducted during pregnancy, the Food and Drug Administration (FDA) has issued pregnancy risk categories (see Table 8-2 and Table 8-3). All commonly used asthma medications are category B or C, but categories do not guarantee safety. It is important to document that informed consent has been obtained from the patient and her partner, to educate the patient and family about medications, and to ensure that risks associated with poorly controlled asthma are clearly understood, because of increased concern of adverse drug reactions during pregnancy (Blaiss, 2004).

Asthma Medication Guidelines

Optimal asthma control must include use of medications but the guiding principle is to use the fewest number of medications possible to control symptoms (Weis, 2003) and to use the drugs with the longest safety records. A joint American College of Allergy, Asthma, and Immunology (ACAAI) and American College of Obstetricians and Gynecologists (ACOG) Committee (2000) incorporated the most recent NAEPP pregnancy guidelines (1993) with specific information available since 1993 on the use of asthma and allergy medications. This report is the most authoritative guide for use of asthma medications during pregnancy to date.

Quick-Relief Medication

The short acting beta$_2$-agonists, albuterol, terbutaline, and metaproterenol, are considered safe during pregnancy. The recommended beta$_2$-agonist has been terbutaline; however new guidelines now recommend inhaled albuterol as the preferred drug (American Academy of Allergy, Asthma and Immunology [AAAAI] 60th Annual Meeting, 2004).

TABLE 8-2: FDA PREGNANCY RISK CATEGORIES (1998)	
Category	**Description**
A	Adequate studies in pregnant women have not demonstrated a risk to the fetus in the first trimester of pregnancy, and there is no risk in later trimesters.
B	Animal studies have not demonstrated a risk to the fetus, but there are no adequate studies in pregnant women. or Animal studies have shown an adverse effect, but adequate studies in pregnant women have not demonstrated a risk to the fetus in the first trimester of pregnancy, and there is no risk later in pregnancy.
C	Animal studies have shown an adverse effect on the fetus, but there are no adequate studies in humans; the benefits from the use of the drug in pregnant women may be acceptable despite its potential risks. or There are no animal reproductive studies and no adequate studies in humans.
D	There is evidence of human fetal risk, but the potential benefits from the use of the drug in pregnant women may be acceptable despite its potential risks.
X	Studies in animals or humans demonstrate fetal abnormalities, or adverse action reports indicate evidence of fetal risk. The risk of use in a pregnant woman clearly outweighs any possible benefit.

Note. Adapted from U.S. Food and Drug Administration (FDA). (2001). *Pregnancy and the drug dilemma.* Retrieved March 12, 2005, from www.fda.gov/fdac/features/2001/301_preg.html

TABLE 8-3: FDA PREGNANCY RISK CATEGORIES FOR ASTHMA MEDICATIONS

Agent	Risk Category
Bronchodilators	
Albuterol	C
Pirbuterol acetate	C
Levalbuterol HCl	C
Salmeterol *serevent*	C
Formoterol fumarate *foradil*	C
Ipratropium bromide *atrovent*	B
Nonsteroidal anti-inflammatory agents	
Cromolyn sodium	B
Nedocromil sodium	B
Leukotriene agents	
Zafirlukast	B
Montelukast sodium	B
Inhaled corticosteroids	
Budesonide *pulmicort*	B
Beclomethasone dipropionate *QVAR*	C
Fluticasone propionate *Flovent*	C
Triamcinolone acetate *azmacort*	C
Flunisolide acetate	C
Fluticasone propionate/salmeterol	C
Oral corticosteroids	C
Theophylline	C
Omalizumab *xolair*	B

Long-acting Beta₂-Agonists

No human data on use of the long-acting beta$_2$-agonist, salmeterol, has been published. Salmeterol is not generally recommended over other beta$_2$-agonists, but it is recommended in patients with moderate to severe asthma who showed good response to this drug before pregnancy (ACOG/ACAAI, 2000).

Long-Term Controller Medication

Inhaled corticosteroids (ICSs) are the long-term controller drugs of choice during pregnancy because they optimize asthma control. Standard doses of ICSs are associated with minimal side effects, and studies that have been conducted show no increase in congenital defects (ACOG/ACAAI,

2000). All ICSs are classified as category C drugs; however, the FDA has recently reclassified budesonide as category B, making this the drug of first choice. Newer ICSs, such as fluticasone are more potent than budesonide but safety data are not available. Because fluticasone does not enter the systemic circulation, it may be continued in women who were well controlled with it before pregnancy (Blaiss, 2004). For patients with moderate persistent asthma that is not adequately controlled by low-dose ICSs, salmeterol as add-on therapy or a medium-dose ICS is recommended. Previous guidelines for cromolyn are no longer recommended. For women with severe persistent asthma, a high-dose ICS, preferably budesonide, and oral prednisone as a last resort at a maximum of 60 mg per day are recommended (AAAAI, 2004).

Oral Corticosteroids

If possible, asthma during pregnancy should be managed without use of systemic steroids because their use has been associated with preterm delivery. Systemic steroids may be needed for severe exacerbations, but the nurse should educate the mother on the signs of preterm labor (Schatz et al., 2004). Other risks are associated with oral corticosteroids, including cleft palate if used in the first trimester, decreased fetal weight gain and preeclampsia when the dosage exceeds 10 mg per day, and worsening of gestational or preexisting diabetes if used long-term (Blaiss, 2004). Severe attacks should be managed aggressively to decrease the risk of fetal hypoxia. The mother should receive quick-relief beta$_2$-agonist via nebulizer, oxygen, and systemic steroids (NHLBI/WHO, 2003).

Other Medication Options

There is no long-term data on the use of leukotriene modifiers during pregnancy. They are generally not recommended (ACOG/ACAAI, 2000). Omalizumab is a new immunoglobulin (Ig) G monoclonal antibody that acts against IgE, one of the major inflammatory mediators in asthma. It is used mainly for severe allergic asthma. The drug has a category B rating but because it is a new drug it should be used cautiously (Blaiss, 2004).

Allergy Medications

Chlorpheniramine and tripelennamine are the recommended antihistamines during pregnancy. If these drugs are not tolerated, cetirizine or loratadine, second-generation antihistamines that have an FDA pregnancy risk category B rating, may be considered after the first trimester (NIH, 2005). Oral decongestants should be avoided in the first trimester. Intranasal steroids can be continued but if initiating treatment, beclomethasone or budesonide are recommended (ACOG/ACAAI, 2000). Likewise, allergen immunotherapy can be safely continued, but not initiated during pregnancy. If immunotherapy is continued, antigen doses should not be increased (Blaiss, 2004).

ANTEPARTUM CARE

Asthma management during the antepartum period begins with a thorough assessment of present symptoms and past asthma severity. Most deaths during pregnancy are associated with underestimation of asthma severity by both patient and physician. In light of these data, new guidelines call for intensive monitoring each month for the duration of the pregnancy. Because of the inaccuracy of subjective assessment, objective measures, such as spirometry and pulse oximetry, must be performed. Baseline pulmonary function tests should be done and repeated each month. Because pregnancy and asthma are associated with breathlessness, objective measures are needed to differentiate its cause. Peak expiratory flow rates remain unchanged during pregnancy and can be accurately used to monitor asthma (Weis, 2003).

Trigger avoidance is critical for optimal asthma control. The mother should receive clear instruction on avoidance of asthma triggers as discussed in chapter 6. Particular attention should be paid to smoking because of its hazardous effect on the developing fetus. Maternal smoking increases the risk of low birth weight by 83%, the risk of preterm delivery by 64%, and the risk of childhood asthma by 25% to 36%. Mothers who smoke are likely to be young, single, and less educated (Jaakkola & Gissler, 2004), and will need support to stop smoking.

INTRAPARTUM CARE

Asthma exacerbations are uncommon during labor (Dombrowski et al, 2004) and there is usually no need to change the asthma medication plan. Peak flows should be measured every 12 hours and fetal monitoring performed. The majority of asthma recommendations during labor call for knowledge of safe medication administration.

If the mother has received systemic corticosteroids for greater than 1 week during pregnancy, she will need intravenous hydrocortisone for possible adrenal suppression. Most of the medications used for preterm labor (magnesium sulfate, nifedipine, or beta-agonists) are safe, but indomethacin may exacerbate asthma and is to be avoided. Labor can safely be induced with oxytocin or one of the prostaglandin E preparations (Weis, 2003).

The best pain control option is epidural anesthesia because it decreases oxygen consumption and enhances response to bronchodilators. Opioids and meperidine are avoided because they are likely to cause bronchospasm. Fentanyl is an alternative to opioids.

If general anesthesia is required, pretreatment with atropine and glycopyrrolate are recommended for their bronchodilator effects. Ketamine is the anesthetic of choice because it reduces airway resistance. Drugs used to treat postpartum hemorrhage need careful selection. Many oxytocic drugs (methylergonovine or ergonovine) cause bronchospasm, but oxytocin may be used (Weis, 2003).

Most women return to their previous asthma severity level within 3 months after delivery (Blaiss, 2004). The mother must understand that it is critical to continue her usual asthma medications. If she elects to breast-feed she should understand that asthma medications are safe (Weis, 2003).

PATIENT EDUCATION

As mentioned earlier, health concerns are heightened during pregnancy. The nurse needs to give the mother opportunity to discuss her fears, particularly concerns about harm to the fetus. The nurse must communicate that optimal health to the fetus is maximized with good asthma management. The goals of asthma management during pregnancy should also be discussed. Other asthma education topics include: safe use of medications, risks associated with undermedication, use of peak flow meters, the effect of pregnancy on the course of asthma, trigger avoidance (with particular emphasis on the hazards of smoking), use of the personal asthma management plan, and safety of breast-feeding while using asthma medications.

SUMMARY

The primary goal of asthma therapy in the child-bearing woman with asthma is to avoid fetal hypoxia because of the devastating effects on the fetus. Normal physiologic changes during pregnancy can have adverse outcomes on the fetus. Current care guidelines call for frequent monitoring of the pregnant woman with asthma. Reduction of use of asthma medication during pregnancy is likely to lead to poor outcomes. Medications should be used to maintain optimal control of asthma. The safety of rescue and controller medications were reviewed as they relate to antepartum and intrapartum care. The nurse can affect positive outcomes by providing mothers with accurate information on asthma goals and safe use of asthma medications.

CASE STUDY

Lily, age 16, has moderate persistent asthma and is 4 weeks pregnant. She is single and has no regular source of medical care. When she is seen in the county health department clinic, she has a nicotine odor but denies smoking. She has wheezing on auscultation and has been experiencing cough in the middle of the night. Her only medication is albuterol and she has used this regularly. She is afraid to take her fluticasone because she thinks it will harm her baby.

Answer the following study questions, writing your responses on a separate sheet of paper. Compare your responses with the answers located at the end of the chapter.

1. What is your priority asthma management concern for Lily?

2. How can Lily's smoking affect her baby?

3. How would you manage Lily's steroid phobia?

4. What recommendation will you make to Lily regarding regular medical care?

Answers to Case Study

1. The priority concern is to help Lily gain control of her asthma. She needs to understand the importance of daily controller medication and regular monitoring by a consistent provider.

2. Lily needs to understand the risk of smoking to her baby. Risks include low birth weight, prematurity, and childhood asthma. Lily fits the smoker profile because she is young, single, and as a 16 year old, probably has not finished high school. She will need extra support and encouragement from the nurse.

3. Lily needs education on the safety of inhaled corticosteroids during pregnancy and risks of uncontrolled asthma. There is more safety data on budesonide than on fluticasone. She may be open to the option of changing her controller medication. Determine if Lily's partner is available for asthma education. Document in the chart that verbal informed consent was given for continuation of the asthma medications. It would be wise to ask Lily if she is able to pay for her medication. Refer her to financial resources if needed.

4. Lily needs to understand that it is important to establish a source of regular medical care and to keep her regularly scheduled appointments each month. Care would ideally be with a specialist because Lily has moderately severe asthma, but this may not be feasible. The nurse should establish a trusting relationship to encourage adherence with regular medical care.

EXAM QUESTIONS

CHAPTER 8
Questions 43-48

43. A woman with mild, persistent asthma wonders how pregnancy will affect her asthma. The nurse should tell the woman

    a. to expect occasional, mild flare-ups.

    b. that mild persistent asthma usually becomes more severe.

    c. that maternal hormones lessen symptoms in women with mild asthma.

    d. that asthma can change. A full assessment is recommended.

44. The greatest danger of undertreatment of asthma during pregnancy is

    a. activity limitation.

    b. fetal hypoxia.

    c. decreased maternal pulmonary function.

    d. increased asthma attacks.

45. In responding to a mother with medication phobia, the nurse should explain that asthma medications have

    a. no effect on maternal outcomes.

    b. no effect on fetal outcomes.

    c. potentially harmful effects.

    d. more benefits than risks.

46. The ICS with the greatest safety profile for use during pregnancy is

    a. beclomethasone.

    b. fluticasone.

    c. budesonide.

    d. cromolyn.

47. The nurse should advise the mother with asthma to seek prenatal care every

    a. week.

    b. 4 weeks.

    c. 6 weeks.

    d. 8 weeks.

48. A woman has received the corticosteroid prednisone on two occasions throughout her pregnancy. The nurse should advise her regarding

    a. risk of birth defects.

    b. signs of preterm labor.

    c. avoiding excessive weight gain.

    d. the need to monitor blood sugar.

REFERENCES

American Academy of Allergy, Asthma and Immunology (AAAAI). (2004, March) *National Asthma Education and Prevention Program Expert Panel Report.* Workshop presented at the 60th Annual Meeting of the AAAAI.

American College of Obstetricians and Gynecologists and the American College of Allergy, Asthma, and Immunology. (2000). Position statement: The use of newer asthma and allergy medications during pregnancy. *Annals of Allergy, Asthma and Immunology, 84,* 475-478.

Blaiss, M. ((2004). Managing asthma during pregnancy: The whys and hows of aggressive control. *Postgraduate Medicine, 115*(5), 55-64.

Dombrowski, M., Schatz, M., Wise, R., Momirova, V., Landon, M., Mabie, W. et al. (2004). Asthma during pregnancy. *Obstetrics & Gynecology, 103,* 5-12.

Gardner, M. & Doyle, N. (2004). Asthma in pregnancy. *Obstetric and Gynecology Clinics, 31*(2). Retrieved September 9, 2004 from, http://home.mdconsultant.com

Jaakkola, J. & Gissler, M. (2004). Maternal smoking in pregnancy, fetal development, and childhood asthma. *American Journal of Public Health, 94,* 136-140.

Kwon, H., Belanger, K., & Bracken, M. (2004). Effect of pregnancy and stage of pregnancy on asthma severity: A systematic review. *American Journal of Obstetrics and Gynecology, 190,* 1201-1210.

National Institutes of Health, National Heart, Lung, and Blood Institute. *National Asthma Education and Prevention Program Working Group on Managing Asthma during Pregnancy: Recommendations for Pharmacologic Treatment – Update 2004.* (2005). (NIH Publication No. 06-3279). Retrieved April 2, 2005, from http://www.nhlib.nih.gov/health/prof/lung/asthma/astpreg.htm

National Institutes of Health/National Heart, Lung, and Blood Institute. (1993). *Management of asthma during pregnancy: Report of the working group on asthma and pregnancy.* (NIH Publication No. 93-3279). Bethesda, MD: National Institutes of Health.

National Heart, Lung, and Blood Institute/World Health Organization. (2003). *Global initiative for asthma: Global strategy for asthma management and prevention.* (NIH Publication No. 02-3659). Retrieved September 12, 2002 from http://www.ginasthma.com

U.S. Food and Drug Administration (FDA). (2001). *Pregnancy and the drug dilemma.* Retrieved March 12, 2005, from www.fda.gov/fdac/features/2001/301_preg.html

Schatz, M., Dombrowski, M., Wise, R., Momirova, V., Landon, M., Mabie, W. et al. (2004). The relationship of asthma medication use to perinatal outcomes. *Journal of Allergy and Clinical Immunology, 113*(6), 1040-1044.

Weis, K.L. (2003). Asthma management across the lifespan: The childbearing woman with asthma. *The Nursing Clinics of North America, 38*(4): 665-673.

CHAPTER 9

THE ADULT AND OLDER ADULT WITH ASTHMA

CHAPTER OBJECTIVE

Upon completion of this chapter, the reader will be able to recognize unique features of asthma in adults and how comorbid conditions and the aging process affect the care of older adults with asthma.

LEARNING OBJECTIVES

After studying this chapter, the reader will be able to

1. identify three features of aspirin induced asthma (AIA) in the adult.

2. recognize three strategies for managing gastroesophageal reflux (GER) in the adult with asthma.

3. recognize the importance of early diagnosis and treatment of work-related asthma (WRA).

4. identify three physiologic changes that complicate asthma care in older adults.

5. identify two ways that comorbid conditions affect asthma care in the older adult.

6. identify five adverse effects of asthma medications in the older adult.

7. recognize three nursing measures that facilitate asthma management in adults and older adults.

OVERVIEW

General aspects of asthma's pathophysiology and management were discussed in chapters 2 through 6. These general concepts apply to the adult and older adult with asthma. Asthma has been considered primarily a disease of children for many years; however, prevalence of asthma is increasing among adults. As more adults present with asthma, our understanding of the disease presentation among these groups increases. The purpose of this chapter is to discuss unique features of asthma primarily seen in these age-groups.

ASPIRIN-INDUCED ASTHMA

In recent years, use of aspirin has increased because it decreases the incidence of myocardial infarction and stroke. Nonsteroidal anti-inflammatory drugs (NSAIDs) are also commonly used, and both aspirin and NSAIDs are usually well tolerated in most people. However, 3% to 20% of adults with asthma experience severe, even fatal reactions after ingestion of these drugs (Szceklik, Sanak, Nizankowska-Mogilnicka, & Kielbasa, 2004). AIA is a distinct clinical syndrome. People who react to aspirin also react to NSAIDs that inhibit cyclo-oxygenase (COX) enzymes (Jenkins, Costello, & Hodge, 2004). AIA is usually first experienced around age 30 and is more common in women.

Once developed, the intolerance remains for life (Szczeklik et al., 2004).

Symptoms begin with intermittent but profuse rhinitis. Later, chronic nasal congestion occurs, often with chronic sinusitis. Nasal polyps are commonly present. Asthma and aspirin intolerance develop 2 to 15 years later (Szczeklik et al., 2004). At the late stage in the illness, a single dose of aspirin or an NSAID causes an acute asthma attack 30 minutes to 3 hours after ingestion (Jenkins et al, 2004). Rhinorrhea, conjunctival irritation, and scarlet flushing of the head and neck commonly accompany the attack. The severity of the reaction depends on the drug potency, dose, and the sensitivity of the person. AIA reactions can be serious and can lead to loss of consciousness, shock, and respiratory arrest.

Persons with AIA have many more times the number of eosinophils (a key cell in the inflammatory process) than those who tolerate aspirin. The high number of eosinophils disrupts the airway epithelium and promotes recruitment of other inflammatory cells into the airway. It is not presently understood how aspirin interacts with inflammatory cells to promote airway constriction (National Heart, Lung, and Blood Institute [NHLBI]/World Health Organization [WHO], 2003).

Many people with asthma are unaware of this syndrome. They may not associate the use of a pain reliever with an asthma attack. Diagnosis of AIA can only be made with certainty by an aspirin challenge. Because of the danger of a severe attack, aspirin challenge must only be conducted in a controlled setting where cardiopulmonary resuscitation can be provided. Patients are challenged when their asthma is under good control and pulmonary functions tests are near normal. Inhalation challenge with lysine-aspirine is safer than an oral aspirin challenge (NHLBI/WHO, 2003). The reaction is considered positive if peak flow or forced expiratory volume in 1 second falls by 15% or more and is accompanied by symptoms of airway obstruction and irritation of the nose and eyes.

Because AIA is present for life, aspirin and all products containing aspirin must be avoided and the patient should wear a Medi-Alert bracelet. It is impossible to predict who will be sensitive to aspirin and NSAIDs; therefore, these drugs are not recommended for any person with asthma (Janson & Roberts, 2003). However, if NSAIDs are needed to treat other conditions, desensitization is possible, but the challenge must be done in a hospital with qualified personnel and resuscitation equipment present (Szczeklik et al., 2004; Jenkins et al., 2004).

Acetominophin is usually well tolerated in patients with AIA at doses less than 1,000 mg (Szczeklik et al., 2004). Although it is premature to recommend COX-2 selective analgesics such as celecoxib, recent studies indicate that patients with AIA tolerate these drugs (Gyllfors et al., 2003). COX-2 inhibitors can be considered with appropriate physician supervision and patient observation for at least 1 hour.

Avoidance of aspirin does not stop the inflammatory progression in patients with AIA. Inhaled corticosteroids continue to be the mainstay of treatment (NHLBI/WHO, 2003).

GASTROESOPHAGEAL REFLUX

Gastroesophageal reflux (GER) is three times more common in people with asthma than in people without asthma. Symptoms include frequent episodes of nocturnal asthma, heartburn, nighttime awakening with acid taste in the mouth, and dyspepsia after meals. Some patients may have no complaints at all. Persons with frequent nocturnal symptoms, despite optimal asthma therapy, and no other complaints should be evaluated for GER. The diagnosis of GER is commonly made based on history, but esophageal pH monitoring with simultaneous pulmonary function testing gives a more accurate diagnosis (NHLBI/WHO, 2003).

GER must be managed to control asthma symptoms. Oral beta-agonists and theophylline should be avoided because they relax the lower esophageal sphincter and increase reflux symptoms. Although not all persons respond to therapy, standard medical treatment for reflux should be prescribed as well as dietary and behavioral modifications. The patient should be taught to eat smaller, more frequent meals and to avoid eating within 3 hours of bedtime. Fatty foods, alcohol, smoking, and caffeine are to be avoided, and the head of the bed should be elevated (NHLBI/WHO, 2003).

The frequent association of GER with asthma has led to the question, "does reflux cause asthma or does asthma cause reflux?" Several physiologic mechanisms have been identified to explain reflux as a cause of asthma; however, recent studies suggest that bronchospasm may trigger reflux (Zerbib et al., 2002). If this is the case, a vicious cycle exists making optimal asthma control even more critical in order to avoid having bronchospasm trigger reflux.

WORK-RELATED ASTHMA

Epidemiology

WRA refers to new onset of asthma as a result of exposure to triggers in the work setting. WRA is different from aggravation of symptoms in a person with previously diagnosed asthma. Approximately 2% to 10% of patients with known asthma experience symptoms as a result of exposure to triggers at work (Zacharisen, 2002). These individuals need to decrease exposure to the irritant and practice good asthma management (Tarlo & Liss, 2003). Approximately 2% to 5% of asthma cases are work-related, that is, are new cases that develop strictly from the workplace. However, WRA may be underreported because of fear of losing one's job or failure to accurately diagnose the illness (Zacharisen, 2002). It is important to distinguish between those with asthma who experience aggravation of symptoms by triggers at work and those with new onset WRA because the method to determine the cause and financial compensation by insurance differs for each (Tarlo & Liss, 2003; Zacharisen, 2002).

Pathophysiology

The pathophysiology of WRA is similar to non-work related asthma and the physiologic response to workplace triggers is similar to the response to allergen or irritant triggers discussed in chapter 6. Most persons with WRA experience immunologically induced symptoms. These individuals are exposed to an agent and experience no immediate symptoms. During this latent period, immunoglobulin (Ig) E is produced. Later exposure to the agent results in asthma symptoms (Tarlo & Liss, 2003; Zacharisen, 2002). Asthma symptoms may begin at work or in the evening after work and improve over weekends and holidays (Tarlo & Liss, 2003). Although less frequent, some WRA is irritant-induced. Symptoms begin within 24 hours of inhalation of large dose of irritants—usually gases, vapors, fumes or particles. Asthma resulting from inhalation of irritants is different from immunologically induced asthma because the airway epithelium is denuded with damage to the submucosa (Zacharisen, 2002).

Risk Factors

Risk factors for WRA include previous history of asthma, history of atopy, (tendency to produce IgE), the nature of the specific agent involved (Zacharisen, 2002), and exposure to environmental tobacco smoke in the workplace (Jaakkola, Piipari, Jaakkola, & Jaakkola, 2003). Persons with atopy usually experience rhinitis and conjunctivitis before the onset of WRA (Zacharisen, 2002).

Hundreds of agents, in a wide variety of work sites, cause WRA. High-risk occupations include farming, painting, cleaning, janitorial work and plastic manufacturing. Examples of causative agents include plants, mold, animal protein, wood dust, chemicals, metals, drugs, flour, enzymes, latex, and irritating cleaning products (Zacharisen, 2002).

Identification of the specific agent is commonly difficult because of multiple exposures in the workplace.

Management

The key to managing WRA is early recognition and referral to a specialist for accurate diagnosis and management. Approximately 50% of patients with WRA improve if they are diagnosed and treated early, but it may take years for pulmonary function tests to show improvement (Zacharisen, 2002). In some patients, especially if the exposure has been over a long period, lung damage is permanent, even after removal from the agent. Prognosis in these patients is poor (Marabini, Siracusa, Stopponi, Tacconi, & Abbritti, 2003).

The diagnostic process may include serial peak flow and symptom recording. The patient records peak flow readings and symptoms four times per day while at work and away from work. Serial recordings are intended to show symptom patterns that may be consistent with work exposure (Tarlo & Liss, 2003). Adherence with peak flow recordings is typically poor. The nurse should use educational and motivational strategies to encourage accurate recording.

Management of WRA is the same as for asthma, but trigger avoidance is critical. Unfortunately, avoidance strategies tend to be expensive. Such strategies include personal respiratory protective equipment, redesign or remediation of the work area, changing departments, or changing occupations (Zacharisen, 2002). Potential for secondary gain related to workmen's compensation exists with WRA. Recent evidence suggests that persons with mild to moderate persistent WRA can remain on the job if they receive treatment with a combination of inhaled corticosteroids (ICSs) and long-acting bronchodilators, reduce exposure to the triggers, and undergo medical surveillance (Marabina et al., 2003).

Role of the Nurse

WRA is a serious condition that can result in permanent lung damage and loss of employment.

The nurse should maintain a high level of suspicion for WRA and encourage early referral to a specialist. The occupational nurse's role may include assisting in identifying agents by visiting the work site, requesting air sampling, assisting in identifying patterns of exposure, promoting a smoke-free work environment, and providing education and emotional support.

CHARACTERISTICS OF ASTHMA IN THE OLDER ADULT

Asthma prevalence, morbidity, and mortality are high in older adults, with highest death rates occurring in those age 65 and older (Centers for Disease Control and prevention, [CDC], 2002). Older adults with asthma experience increased day and nighttime symptoms that persist for longer durations than in any other age-group. Asthma related hospitalizations in this group are more common and tend to be prolonged (Janson & Roberts, 2003).

Asthma is commonly undertreated or undiagnosed in the elderly (Braman, 2003). This is unfortunate because untreated asthma significantly alters quality of life and leads to excessive use of healthcare. Of all age-groups, asthma is probably most difficult to diagnose and treat in the older adult. Many reasons contribute to this difficulty: (a) declining lung function (Zeleznik, 2003), (b) comorbid conditions, (c) poor symptom perception, (d) difficulty performing lung function tests (NHLBI/WHO, 2003), (e) increase in adverse medication effects, (f) complex medication regimes (National Asthma Education and Prevention Program [NAEPP], 1997), and (g) sensory impairment (NAEPP, 1996). These difficulties coupled with memory loss and limited financial resources lead to high rates of nonadherence to asthma treatment in older adults (Braman, 2003).

Normal Aging of the Respiratory System

The normal process of aging produces decline in lung function. Age-related changes include:

- altered composition of airway immune cells

- decreases in collagen content in the lung with reduced airway diameter on expiration

- emphysematous changes

- decreased pulmonary muscle strength

- declining pulmonary function

- decreased sensation of dyspnea

- lower arterial partial pressure of oxygen

- changes to the pharmacologic stimulation of bronchial smooth muscle (Zeleznik, 2003).

These changes do not affect day-to-day activities of most older adults, but they do become a factor when illness stresses limited oxygen reserves (Zeleznik, 2003). For the older adult with asthma, these changes increase the risk of lower respiratory tract infections and airway obstruction. The changes also make it difficult to perform pulmonary function tests and recognize asthma symptoms and reduce the patient's response to beta-agonists.

Diagnosis of Asthma

Asthma in the older adult may be preexisting or newly acquired following a serious respiratory infection (Braman, 2003). New-onset asthma is commonly misdiagnosed or may be confused with chronic obstructive pulmonary disease (COPD), congestive heart failure, or GER. It may also be attributed to normal aging or simply ignored (Braman, 2003). Left ventricular failure, or "cardiac asthma" can produce episodes of wheezing, dyspnea, and cough that mimic asthma and confuse the clinical picture. Some older adults expect dyspnea on exertion because of declining activity levels and lack of physical fitness. Some may attribute chronic cough to smoking. Others have diminished perception of dyspnea or limited financial resources and fail to seek care (NAEPP, 1996).

The gold standard for diagnosing asthma is to demonstrate reversibility of airway obstruction after administration of beta-agonists. Older adults may fail to respond to bronchodilators, especially if the disease has been long standing. A 2-week course of oral steroids may be needed to demonstrate reversibility (NAEPP, 1996). The best diagnostic test is spirometry, but this test is often underused, perhaps because older adults have difficulty performing the maneuver. Baseline spirometry should be performed and repeated every 3 to 6 months. Lung function testing is especially critical because of reduced perception of dyspnea (Braman, 2003).

Goals of Therapy

The goals of asthma therapy in the older adult are essentially the same as in other groups. Specific goals include:

- recognizing and treating exacerbations promptly

- avoiding aggravating other comorbid conditions

- minimizing adverse drug reactions

- optimizing activity level and quality of life (NAEPP, 1996).

Goals may be more difficult to achieve in the older adult. The nurse should provide education to raise expectations from treatment as high as possible (NAEPP, 1996).

Triggers

Sensitivity to allergens declines in older adults (NAEPP, 1996); however, avoidance of allergens is still recommended (Braman, 2003). The most common triggers are upper respiratory tract infections, medications used to treat other conditions (NAEPP, 1996) and irritants such as smoke, paint, and varnish (Braman, 2003). The usual trigger avoidance measures should be taught. These measures include an annual flu shot and periodic pneumococcal vaccine administration (NAEPP, 1996).

Pharmacologic Management

Asthma Management

Pharmacologic management is particularly challenging in the older adult. Most older adults with asthma need continuous asthma treatment programs (Braman, 2003) and frequent monitoring because side effects are common.

Beta$_2$-agonists can cause electrocardiogram changes, hypokalemia, tremor, and hypoxemia. Persons with cardiac disease or on high-dose beta$_2$-agonists may need continuous cardiac monitoring. Oral beta-agonists should be avoided because they may cause tremor and increased heart rate and blood pressure (NAEPP, 1996). As mentioned earlier, beta$_2$-agonist response declines with age, but the anticholinergic response remains intact. The older adult may experience greater bronchodilation from the anticholinergic drug ipratropium with less tremor and arrhythmia (NAEPP, 1996).

ICSs are the preferred treatment in older adults, but high doses (more than 1,000 mcg/day) are associated with increased dermal thinning, bruising, and osteoporosis. Calcium and vitamin D are recommended as well as monitoring with bone density tests (NAEPP, 1996). The nurse should stress the importance of adhering to ICS therapy because one of the goals of therapy is to avoid use of systemic steroids. Use of systemic steroids increases the risk of common complications in older adults, such as diabetes, osteoporosis, hypertension, cataracts, depressed immunity and mood swings (Braman, 2003). In addition, systemic steroid clearance is slow in older adults. The nurse must monitor for electrolyte imbalances—especially hypokalemia—hypertension, and hyperglycemia, worsening glaucoma, and aggravation of gastric and peptic ulcers. Systemic steroids can also increase depression, and depression usually results in increased adherence problems (NAEPP, 1996).

Data on the use of leukotriene modifying agents in older adults are limited. They are effective in exercise-induced asthma and allergen induced asthma, conditions not relevant to the older adult. Leukotriene modifying agents are generally safe, but they are not preferred over low-dose ICSs (Braman, 2003). Theophylline has many side effects and drug interactions; therefore, its use in older adults has declined in recent years (Braman, 2003).

Drug Interactions with Nonasthma Medications

As mentioned above, comorbid conditions are common in the older adult. Care must be taken to avoid adverse drug interaction with medications used to treat other conditions. Table 9-1 lists commonly used nonasthma drugs and their potential adverse effects on asthma.

Beta-blockers cause bronchospasm and should be avoided. Contents of eye drops need to be checked and avoided if they contain a beta-blocker. Diuretics that do not spare potassium (i.e., thiazides) cause a significant drop in potassium and magnesium if taken with beta-agonists, especially if digitalis is also being taken (NAEPP, 1996).

Nursing Care

Education is a major component of asthma management for the older adult. The nurse should actively involve other family members and seek feedback to affirm understanding. COPD is easily confused with asthma and differences need to be specifically clarified (NAEPP, 1996), although frequently both conditions coexist. Because perception of dyspnea is decreased in older adults, the nurse should encourage use of a peak flow meter or symptom diary. The importance of recognizing early warning signs and prompt treatment must be stressed.

Medication errors are common in older adults. The older adult needs more memory aids and visual enhancements for accurate medication administration. Medications may have to be color coded and coordinated with color coding on personal asthma self-management plans. Hand strength and

TABLE 9-1: NONASTHMA MEDICATIONS WITH INCREASED POTENTIAL FOR ADVERSE EFFECTS IN THE OLDER ADULT WITH ASTHMA

Medication	Comorbid Condition	Adverse Effect
Beta-adrenergic blocking agents	Hypertension Heart disease Tremor Glaucoma	• Worsening asthma • Bronchospasm • Beta response to bronchodilator • Beta response to epinephrine in anaphylaxis
Nonsteroidal anti-inflammatory drugs	Arthritis Musculoskeletal diseases	• Worsening asthma • Bronchospasm
Nonpotassium sparing diuretics	Hypertension Congestive heart failure	• Worsening cardiac function/ arrhythmias due to hypokalemia
Angiotensin-converting enzyme inhibitors	Heart failure Hypertension	• Increased cough
Cholinergic agents	Urinary retention Glaucoma	• Bronchospasm • Bronchorrhea
Certain nonsedating antihistamines	Allergic rhinitis	• Worsening cardiac function/ventricular arrhythmias due to prolonged QTc interval

Note. From National Asthma Education and Prevention Program. (1996) *Working group report: Considerations for diagnosing asthma in the elderly.* (NIH, Publication No. 96-3662).

inspiratory flow are needed to actuate asthma medication devices. Metered-dose inhaler (MDI) and dry powder inhaler (DPI) techniques need to be taught carefully, evaluated, and frequently reviewed. Spacers increase accurate delivery with MDIs, but drug delivery for the older adult is probably best with DPIs (NAEPP, 1996).

Some older adults become homebound because of their dependence on nebulizers (Janson & Roberts, 2003). New lightweight, handheld nebulizers are available and easily carried. Although expensive, these nebulizers may be ideal for persons who have become homebound. (See the resources for manufacturers of handheld nebulizers). The nurse should assess the older adult's ability to purchase asthma medications and devices. Referrals to appropriate agencies or programs should be made as needed.

The nurse should recognize that multiple complex regimes, memory decline, hearing and vision problems, altered sleep, and depression in the older adult contribute to poor adherence to asthma therapy. Older adults need more time for explanations of care, more frequent review of use of asthma devices, and a written personal management plan. The management plan must be detailed and written in large print. The plan must include what to do for asthma flare-ups and when to call the provider (NAEPP, 1996).

CASE STUDY

Mrs. Smith, age 78, visits the geriatric care clinic. She is being treated with propranolol and diuril for hypertension, chlorpropamide for type 2 diabetes, and takes ibuprofen for joint pain. She was recently diagnosed with asthma and placed on albuterol, 2 puffs every 4 hours as needed, and fluticasone, 110 mcg/puff, 2 puffs twice daily. During the history, Mrs. Smith appears confused. She states that she has trouble remembering, but thinks she takes the albuterol twice daily and uses the fluticasone as needed. She has no written management plan and no spacer. She reports nocturnal cough almost every night, but states, "That's to be expected at my age." She lives by herself, but a daughter who lives nearby looks in on her frequently. She is presently having difficulty breathing and has audible wheezes.

Answer the following case study questions, writing your responses on a separate sheet of paper. Compare your responses with the answers at the end of the chapter.

1. What are the asthma management goals for Mrs. Smith?

2. What nonasthma medications place Mrs. Smith at risk for worsening asthma?

3. How does Mrs. Smith's mental status and perception affect her self-management?

4. What resource should the nurse include in the plan of care?

5. What would the ideal written self-management plan for Mrs. Smith look like?

Answers to Case Study

1. The goals for Mrs. Smith include minimizing adverse drug reactions with nonasthma medications; preventing nocturnal symptoms, educating her regarding proper use of asthma medications and use of a spacer or DPI, recognizing and treating asthma symptoms early, and avoiding aggravation of her diabetes, hypertension, and arthritis.

2. Propranolol, diuril, and ibuprofen place Mrs. Smith at risk for worsening asthma. Propranolol is a beta-blocker and causes bronchospasm. The nurse should recognize this and ask the physician if there is another class of hypertensive medication that would effectively control Mrs. Smith's blood pressure. Diuril is a nonpotassium-sparing diuretic and would cause significant drops in potassium and magnesium if taken with beta$_2$-agonists. Mrs. Smith is using her albuterol, a beta$_2$-agonist, excessively. She is at risk for electrolyte imbal-

ance. The ibuprofen could worsen asthma. Mrs. Smith may tolerate celecoxib, but she should discuss long-term side effects of this drug with her primary careprovider.

3. Mrs. Smith has a complex medical regimen that is difficult to follow. Her memory loss and perception that outcomes caused by poor asthma management are inevitable because of her age complicate management of and adherence to treatment.

4. Mrs. Smith's daughter should be asked to accompany Mrs. Smith to clinic and be included in the education plan. A clearly written asthma management plan with memory aids such as medication color codes should be developed and reviewed with Mrs. Smith and her daughter.

5. The ideal self-management plan would include a minimum number of medications once or twice daily. Mrs. Smith's response to albuterol should be assessed. She may experience more relief with ipratropium, and because this drug is not a beta$_2$-agonist, it would not interact with diuril. Mrs. Smith needs focused education on the use of rescue versus controller medication. Every effort should be made to increase adherence with the fluticasone because further deterioration would require treatment with oral steroids. Mrs. Smith needs a spacer, and her MDI technique needs to be assessed. Fluticasone is available in a DPI, which may improve drug delivery for Mrs. Smith. Finally, Mrs. Smith needs to have her early warning signs clearly identified. She needs to be encouraged to notice these signs and log them into a daily symptom diary or use a peak flow meter if she is able. Clear indications for calling her primary care provider need to be written.

EXAM QUESTIONS

CHAPTER 9
Questions 49-55

49. Symptoms indicating that a person with asthma is experiencing an aspirin-induced reaction include

    a. runny nose, reddening of the face, and reddened eyes.

    b. generalized body rash, intense itching, and air hunger.

    c. severe retracting, diaphoresis, urticaria rash.

    d. pale, clammy skin and swollen lips.

50. The nurse should instruct the adult with asthma and GER to

    a. change from the inhaled form to the oral form of albuterol.

    b. avoid eating for three hours upon rising in the morning.

    c. eat large, well spaced meals.

    d. avoid fatty foods, caffeine, alcohol, and smoking.

51. Consequences of delayed treatment of long-term work-related asthma (WRA) include

    a. permanent lung damage.

    b. transient lung damage.

    c. intense rhinitis.

    d. restrictive lung disease.

52. Physiologic lung changes in the older adult that affect asthma care include

    a. altered composition of airway immune cells.

    b. increased collagen in the airways.

    c. exaggerated reaction of airway smooth muscle to beta$_2$-agonists.

    d. heightened sensation of dyspnea.

53. Comorbid conditions affect asthma care by

    a. increasing the risk of adverse drug reactions.

    b. presenting a well defined symptom pattern.

    c. increasing resistance to controller medication.

    d. increasing the older adult's adherence to medication.

54. The class of drugs that worsen bronchospasm and decrease the bronchodilator effect of rescue medication is the

    a. beta$_2$-agonists.

    b. beta-blockers.

    c. NSAIDs.

    d. ACE inhibitors.

55. A nursing measure that facilitates asthma management for the older adult is

    a. focusing all teaching toward a family member.

    b. limiting disease explanations because it will confuse the older adult.

    c. providing a management plan with specific steps clearly written.

    d. teaching the older adult that COPD and asthma are similar.

REFERENCES

Braman, S. (2003). Asthma in the elderly. *Clinics in Geriatric Medicine, 19*(1). Retrieved August 9, 2004 from http://home.mdconsult.com/das/article/body/39766891-2/jorg=journal&source

Centers for Disease Control and Prevention. (2002). Surveillance for asthma — United States, 1980–1999. *Morbidity and Mortality Weekly Report, 51*(SS-1), 1-13.

Gyllfors, P., Bochenek, G., Overholt, M., Drupka, D., Kumlin, M., Sheller, J., et al. (2003). Biochemical and clinical evidence that aspirin-intolerant asthmatic subjects tolerate the cyclo-oxygenase 2-selective analgesic drug celecoxib. *Journal of Allergy and Clinical Immunology, 111*, 1116-1121.

Jaakkola, M., Piipari, R., Jaakkola, N., & Jaakkola, J. (2003). Environmental tobacco smoke and adult-onset asthma: A population-based incident case-control study. *American Journal of Public Health, 93*(12), 2055 - 2059.

Janson, S. & Roberts, J. (2003). Asthma management across the lifespan: Applications for the adult and older adult. *Nursing Clinics of North America, 38*(4), 675-687.

Jenkins, C., Costello, J., & Hodge, L. (2004). Systematic review of prevalence of aspirin induced asthma and its implications for clinical practice. *British Medical Journal, 328*(7437), 434-445.

Maghni, K., Lemiere, C., Ghezzo, H, Yuquan, W., & Malo, J. (2004). Airway inflammation after cessation of exposure to agents causing occupational asthma. *American Journal of Respiratory and Critical Care Medicine, 169*, 367-372.

Marabini, A., Siracusa, A., Stopponi, R., Tacconi, C., & Abritti, G. (2003). Outcomes of occupational asthma in patients with continuous exposure. *Chest, 124*, 2372-2376.

National Asthma Education and Prevention Program. (1996). *Working group report: Considerations for diagnosing and managing asthma in the elderly.* (NIH, Publication No. 96-3662).

National Heart, Lung, and Blood Institute/World Health Organization. (2003). *Global initiative for asthma: Global strategies for asthma management and prevention.* (NIH Publication No. 02-3659). Retrieved September 12, 2002, from http://www.ginasthma.com

Szczeklik, A., Sanak, M., Nizankowska-Mogilnicka, E., & Kielbasa, B. (2004). Aspirin intolerance and the cyclooxygenase-leukotriene pathways. *Current Opinion in Pulmonary Medicine, 10*(1), 51-56.

Tarlo, S. & Liss, G. (2003). Occupational asthma: An approach to diagnosis and management. *Canadian Medical Association Journal, 168*(7), 867-871.

Zacharisen, M. (2002). Occupational asthma. *Medical Clinics of North America, 86*(5), Retrieved August 19, 2004, from http://home.mdconsult.com/das/article/body/40046897-2/jorg=journal&source=MI&sp-12

Zeleznik, J. (2003). Normative aging of the respiratory system. *Clinics in Geriatric Medicine, 19*(1). Retrieved August 9, 2004, from http://home.mdconsult.com/das/article/body/39766891-2/jorg=journal&source

Zerbib, F., Guisset, O., Lamouliatte, H., Quinton, A., Galmiche, J., & Tunon-de-Lara, J. (2002). Effects of bronchial obstruction on lower esophageal sphincter motility and gastroesophageal reflux in patients with asthma. *American Journal of Respiratory and Critical Care Medicine, 166,* 1206-1211.

CHAPTER 10

ACUTE ASTHMA MANAGEMENT

CHAPTER OBJECTIVE

Upon completion of this chapter, the reader will be able to recognize signs and symptoms of an acute asthma attack and apply appropriate nursing interventions.

LEARNING OBJECTIVES

After studying this chapter, the reader will be able to

1. recognize three signs of an acute asthma attack.

2. recognize three characteristics that distinguish mild, moderate, and severe asthma attacks.

3. identify three interventions for management of an acute attack at home.

4. identify five characteristics of a person with near-fatal asthma.

5. identify three nursing interventions for the person presenting with asthma in the emergency room (ER).

6. recognize three patient education topics specific to the ER.

7. identify three nursing interventions for the hospitalized person with asthma.

OVERVIEW

General aspects of asthma management and treatment applications across the lifespan have been discussed in previous chapters. This chapter focuses on management of the person with an acute asthma attack at home, in the ER, or in the hospital. Hospitalizations and ER visits are preventable because asthma is a controllable disease. The nurse should recognize the importance of providing education to patients in the ER or hospital setting because attacks severe enough to result in ER visits or hospitalizations indicate poor asthma control.

ACUTE ASTHMA ATTACKS

Characteristics of Acute Asthma Attacks

Asthma attacks are episodes of rapidly progressive cough, shortness of breath, wheezing, tight chest, or some combination of these symptoms (National Heart, Lung, and Blood Institute [NHLBI]/World Health Organization [WHO], 2003). However, not all of these symptoms may manifest in each person with asthma. Wheezing is the symptom most commonly associated with asthma; however, some people with asthma never wheeze; rather, they experience cough as their primary symptom. These individuals are said to have cough variant asthma. Failure to recognize this presentation of asthma has resulted in underdiagnosis and undertreatment.

Respiratory distress, which commonly accompanies acute attacks, is characterized by difficulty exhaling air. This difficulty is measurable

(NHLBI/WHO, 2003). The nurse may note a prolonged expiration compared to inspiration when auscultating the lungs and a drop in peak flow rate.

Severity of Attacks

Asthma attacks range in severity from mild to severe to, occasionally, life-threatening. Attacks usually develop over a number of hours to days but can occur in minutes. A viral upper respiratory tract infection (URI) or allergen commonly triggers the acute attack, but a gradual pattern of deterioration usually reflects poor adherence to the asthma management plan (NHLBI/WHO, 2003).

The severity of the attack must be assessed because treatment is based on severity. Attacks are classified as mild, moderate or severe. See Table 10-1 for assessment parameters used to rate attack severity. Note that wheezing is not an accurate indicator of airway obstruction. In fact, absence of wheezing is an indicator of impending respiratory arrest because no air is moving to create the wheeze (Corbridge & Corbridge, 2004).

There are several unique assessment parameters in children. Although accurate in adults, pulsus paradoxus (when the pulse becomes weaker during inspiration) is inaccurate in children and therefore is usually not measured in children. Oxygen saturation (O_2 sat), on the other hand, is especially important in children because pulmonary function is hard to obtain in this age-group. O_2 sats are usually above 95% in children. A value of less than 92% indicates need for hospital admission. Although respiratory failure is rare in infants, they must be monitored closely because anatomical differences in the developing airway place them at risk. Breathlessness severe enough to prevent feeding in an infant is a sign of impending respiratory failure.

Arterial blood gases are not routinely recommended unless a peak flow of less than 50% is predicted or the patient does not respond to treatment (NHLBI/WHO, 2003).

Recognition and Recovery from Attacks

It is critical to recognize and treat symptoms promptly. Failure to do so results in increased morbidity and mortality (NHLBI/WHO, 2003). A key goal of asthma education is that the learner will recognize early warning signs and symptoms. However, persons with asthma are known to vary greatly in their ability to recognize early warning signs and symptoms. Some individuals report no symptoms despite significant decline in lung function. This so-called "poor perception" of airway obstruction appears to be more common in males and in those with long- standing asthma and may represent an adaptation response. An adaptation response is when a person lives with asthma for so long that he or she gets used to having obstruction and forgets what it feels like to have an open airway. This is dangerous because the person then fails to recognize impending attacks. It is a risk factor for fatal asthma.

Recovery from attacks is gradual. It may take many days for pulmonary functions to return to normal and weeks for airway hyperresponsiveness to decrease. Unfortunately, symptoms are not accurate indicators of improvement. The patient needs to be instructed to continue treatment until objective test results return to normal (NHLBI/WHO, 2003).

ACUTE CARE MANAGEMENT IN THE HOME

The principle that guides acute asthma management is recognition of symptoms and treatment of the exacerbation as quickly as possible. Therapy treatment for the attack should start at home. Teaching patients to make treatment decisions is empowering and gives a sense of control. The degree of decision making depends on several factors: experience and availability of the healthcare provider, the patient's experience, the availability of

TABLE 10-1: CLASSIFYING SEVERITY OF ASTHMA EXACERBATIONS

	Mild	**Moderate**	**Severe**	**Impending Respiratory Arrest**
SYMPTOMS				
Breathlessness	Walking	Talking (infant – softer, shorter cry; difficulty feeding)	At rest (infant – stops feeding)	
Positioning	Can lie down	Prefers sitting	Sits upright	
Talks in	Sentences	Phrases	Words	
Alertness	May be agitated	Usually agitated	Usually agitated	Drowsy or confused
SIGNS				
Respiratory rate	Increased	Increased	Often > 30/min	
	Guide to rates of breathing in awake children Age — Normal rate < 2 months — < 60/minute 2–12 months — < 50/minute 1–5 years — < 40/minute 6–8 years — < 30/minute			
Use of accessory muscles	Usually not	Commonly	Usually	Paradoxical thoraco-abdominal movement
Wheeze	Moderate Often only end expiratory	Loud through-out exhalation	Usually loud throughout inhalation and exhalation	Absent
Pulse/minute	< 100	100–120	> 120	Bradycardia
	Guide to normal pulse rates in children Age — Normal rate 2–12 months — < 160/minute 1–2 years — < 120/minute 2–8 years — < 110/minute			
Pulsus paradoxus	Absent < 10 mm Hg	May be present 10 - 25 mm Hg	Often present > 25 mm Hg (adult) 20-40 mm Hg (child)	Absence suggests respiratory muscle fatigue
FUNCTIONAL ASSESSMENT				
PEFR % predicted or % personal best	80%	Approx. 50%-80%	< 50% predicted or personal best or response lasts < 2hrs	
PaO_2 (on air)	Normal	> 60 mm Hg	< 60 mm Hg Possible cyanosis	
PCO_2	< 42 mm Hg	< 42 mm Hg	$\geq$ 42 mm Hg; possible respiratory failure	
SaO_2% (on air) at sea level	> 95%	91-95%	< 91%	

Note. Presence of several parameters, but not necessarily all, indicates the general classification of the exacerbation. This is a general guide only. Many of the parameters have not been studied.

Note. From National Asthma Education and Prevention Program. (1997). Export panel report 2. *Guidelines for the diagnosis and management of asthma.* (NIH Publication No. 97-4051) Bethesda, MD: National Institutes of Health, National Heart, Lung, and Blood Institute. Available online at www.nhlbi.nih.gov/guidelines/asthma/asthgdln.pdf

medications and a written action plan detailing treatment steps (NHLBI/WHO, 2003).

Regardless of setting, peak flow monitoring is an integral part of the treatment plan. Peak flow is a guide to therapy because patients and physicians tend to underestimate the severity of obstruction. However, clinical judgment should be used in obtaining readings in the severely dyspneic person because measuring peak flow can worsen bronchospasm (Corbridge & Corbridge, 2004).

Initial acute treatment consists of administration of rapid acting bronchodilators, 2 to 4 puffs every 20 minutes for the first hour. After the first hour, the dose depends upon the severity of the attack. Mild attacks are treated with 2 to 4 puffs of rapid-acting bronchodilator with a spacer. Moderate attacks are treated with 6 to 10 puffs every 1-2 hours, and severe attacks with up to 10 puffs or nebulized bronchodilator at intervals less than 1 hour. No additional treatment is needed if the peak flow returns to 80% of predicted or better for 3 to 4 hours (NHLBI/WHO, 2003).

Limited studies indicate a benefit to increasing the inhaled corticosteroid (ICS) dose early in the recovery phase (NHLBI/WHO, 2003). Patients are commonly advised to double the ICS dose; however, this recommendation lacks supporting evidence. Higher doses may be appropriate but the optimal dose has not been determined.

Alternatively, oral corticosteroids in the amount of 1 to 2 mg/kg/day up to 60 mg/day may be given in all but the mildest of attacks to speed recovery. If improvement is sustained, the patient may continue care at home, with consultation. It bears repeating that full recovery is gradual. Medications will need to be continued for several days. It should also be kept in mind that even people with mild asthma can have sudden severe attacks.

Some patients fail to respond completely to treatment at home. Patients should be referred to the ER if they continue to deteriorate, show no improvement 2 to 6 hours after steroid administration, fail to respond promptly and sustain a response for at least 3 hours, demonstrate a peak flow of < 60% after bronchodilator treatment, or are at high risk for death (NHLBI/WHO, 2003).

The Fatality Prone Profile

Approximately 1.1% to 7% of patients die from asthma attacks. To prevent death, it is important to identify those at risk (Magadle, Berar-Yanay, & Weiner, 2002). These patients share distinct characteristics that the nurse should recognize. The fatality-prone profile is listed in Table 10-2.

TABLE 10-2: FATALITY PRONE CHARACTERISTICS

- History of a near-fatal attack that required intubation
- Hospitalization or emergency room visit in the last year
- Current or recent use of oral corticosteroids
- Lack of current inhaled corticosteroid use
- Overreliance on beta$_2$-agonist, especially more than one canister/month
- Nonadherence to the asthma management plan
- History of psychiatric or psychosocial problems

(NHLBI/WHO, 2003)

In addition, those with near-fatal asthma tend to have more severe disease. They report increase use of medication in the past 12 months and report frequent symptoms, especially nocturnal cough, despite increased medication use. They report significantly more allergy and eczema and commonly give a history of food allergies with life-threatening reaction. These patients are also more likely to smoke. Most people with asthma suffer attacks triggered by URIs or exercise, but people with near-fatal asthma are more likely to report emotional events as triggering the attack (Mitchell, Tough, Semple, Green, & Hessel, 2002). These patients should be immediately referred to the ER and receive intensive education and long-term follow up.

Near-fatal asthma may not be disturbing to the patient because perception of dyspnea is typically poor, especially if asthma is of long duration. Ability to perceive dyspnea is important because it is the most important indicator to the patient for making treatment decisions. Poor perception places patients at increased risk for death because they typically undertreat themselves (Magadle, Berar-Yanay, & Weiner, 2002). The nurse should question patients about their perception of dyspnea and correlate their responses with a peak flow reading as a more objective assessment. These patients should be counseled to use a peak flow meter regularly.

MANAGEMENT IN THE ER

Goals of Care

Despite the asthma management goal of no ER or hospital visits, there are approximately 1.8 million asthma-related ER visits annually in the United States and 500,000 asthma-related hospitalizations (Silverman, Osborn, Runge, Gallagher, Chiang, Feldman et al., 2002). The primary goal of ER treatment is to promptly treat the exacerbation, identify the triggering event, educate to prevent recurrence, and refer for further education and follow-up care.

Assessment is important but it should not delay treatment. A history should be obtained and physical examination should be performed as treatment is started. The history includes exercise tolerance and nocturnal symptoms, all current medications and dosages, medications given to treat the current attack and the patient's response, cause of the present attack, and near-fatal risk factors—especially perception of dyspnea and prior hospitalization, intubation, ER visits, or intensive care admissions (NHLBI/WHO, 2003).

Assessment includes pulse oximetry, spirometry, and peak flow monitoring. Although recommended by national asthma guidelines (NAEPP, 1997), peak flow monitoring may be difficult to obtain in children presenting to the ER. Children who are not followed by a specialist are commonly unfamiliar with the maneuver, and severe airway obstruction may make taking the maximal inhalation required for accurate peak flow readings impossible (Gorelick, Stevens, Schultz, & Scribano, 2004).

Therapy

Oxygen is administered with the goal of raising oxygen saturation to 90% in adults or 95% in children. Oxygen is titrated according to pulse oximetry (NHLBI/WHO, 2003). Recent data suggest that dehydration, a known trigger in exercise-induced asthma, is a factor in patients presenting to the ER with severe exacerbation. Because dehydration alone may cause bronchoconstriction, all inspired oxygen should be humidified (Moloney, O'Sullivan, Hogan, Poulter, & Burke, 2002).

Rapid-acting beta$_2$-agonists are administered via nebulizers in children; however, metered-dose inhaler (MDI) delivery is preferred in adults because it is equivalent to nebulized administration but is quicker and easier to administer and has fewer side effects. According to national guidelines, intravenous (IV) beta$_2$-agonists may be added if the patient fails to respond to high-dose or continuous nebulizer treatments, but the patient should be closely monitored for toxicity (NHLBI/WHO, 2003). However, recent data from multiple studies identified no supporting evidence for the use of the IV route and recommended that all beta$_2$-agonists be given via inhalation (Travers, et al., 2001). Patients with severe airway obstruction may benefit from continuous (four nebulized treatments/hour) beta$_2$-agonist administration early in the ER treatment (Camargo, Spooner, & Rowe, 2003).

Levalbuterol is an isomer of albuterol that has the therapeutic effects of the parent drug with none of the side effects. Its use as the initial therapy for acute asthma is being studied because it produces faster and greater bronchodilatation than albuterol. Children treated with levalbuterol had lower hospitalization rates than those treated with albuterol (Corbridge & Corbridge, 2004).

Systemic steroids speed recovery and are an integral part of therapy in all but the mildest attacks (NHLBI/WHO, 2003). As a standard of care, systemic steroids should be administered within 1 hour of presentation to the ER. Prompt administration of systemic steroids reduces the need for hospitalization (Rowe, Spooner, Ducharme, Bretzlaff, & Bota, 2001). The oral route of administration is preferred because it is noninvasive and inexpensive. If vomiting occurs, the same dose is administered IV. Clinical improvement is expected within 4 to 6 hours.

ALTERNATIVE THERAPEUTIC MANAGEMENT OPTIONS IN THE ER SETTING

Epinephrine

Epinephrine is usually reserved for anaphylaxis or angioedema, but it can be used in asthma if beta$_2$-agonists are not available. Adverse effects are common with epinephrine administration, especially in the patient who is hypoxic (NHLBI/WHO, 2003).

Aminophylline

Aminophylline was commonly administered as a first-line drug for acute asthma in the past. Current data indicate that aminophylline does not give additional bronchodilation compared with standard beta$_2$-agonists. Because no group was identified that benefitted from aminophylline, and because it is associated with cardiac arrhythmia and vomiting,

it is no longer recommended (Parameswaran, Belda, & Rowe, 2000).

Heliox

Heliox is a blend of helium and oxygen. When given in combination with nebulized albuterol, it provides more effective bronchodilation and improved pulmonary function in adult patients with severe asthma. Heliox decreases airway resistance and decreases the work of breathing. It is administered via a high-flow, nonrebreathing delivery system (Kress, et al., 2002).

Magnesium Sulfate

Magnesium sulfate is a bronchodilator that may be useful in adults with severe asthma or in adults and children who fail to respond to initial treatment. It is usually given as a 2-gram infusion. There is no need for additional monitoring because this is a safe drug (NHLBI/WHO, 2003). Patients may experience flushing, light-headedness, lethargy, nausea, or burning at the IV site. In a large multicenter study, patients with the most severe respiratory compromise showed improvement. Those with less severe asthma showed no benefit (Silverman, et al., 2002).

Ipratropium Bromide

Ipratropium bromide is an anticholinergic drug that blocks bronchoconstriction by the cholinergic pathway. It is administered by inhalation and is poorly absorbed by the systemic circulation; therefore, there are very few or no side effects. Because its onset of action is 3 to 30 minutes, it is suitable as a rescue medication. It peaks in 1 to 2 hours and its duration of action is 6 hours. Because its site of action is different than albuterol, it may be given in combination to give better bronchodilation. It is indicated for children and adults with severe exacerbation, but it must be given in multiple doses to achieve the desired effect (Rodrigo & Rodrigo, 2002; Plotnick & Ducharme, 2000).

Antibiotics

Asthma exacerbations are commonly associated with clinical signs of infection such as purulent sputum or nasal discharge. These infections are usually viral. Ambiguous clinical signs and the belief that mucus plugging places the patient at increased risk for infection has led to frequent and inappropriate use of antibiotics for acute asthma. Antibiotics are not recommended for the treatment of acute attacks, except as needed for concurrent infections such as sinusitis or pneumonia (National Asthma Education and Prevention Program [NAEPP], 2003).

PRIORITY ASTHMA EDUCATION TOPICS IN THE ER SETTING

Criteria for Discharge

The patient who has a peak flow of 40% to 60% and improved pulmonary function is a candidate for discharge from the ER if adherence and follow-up guidelines can be met (NHLBI, 2002), although some recommend a peak flow of 70% or more as criteria for discharge (Corbridge & Corbridge, 2004). Discharge recommendations include a 5 to 7 day course of oral corticosteroids, continued ICS therapy, and continued but tapered use of a beta$_2$-agonist over several days until symptoms and peak flow measurements improve. Because the patient is discharged on around-the-clock beta$_2$-agonists, usual doses of long-acting beta$_2$-agonists should be temporarily discontinued (NHLBI/WHO, 2003).

Nursing Implications

Acute asthma attacks that result in hospitalization commonly result from poor asthma management, especially in those patients who use the ER for crisis management. These patients tend to have a poor understanding of asthma and of the need for daily controller medication (Corbridge & Corbridge, 2004). Patients using the ER tend to rely solely on rapid-acting beta$_2$-agonists and oral corticosteroids for rescue management. As many as 75% of patients visiting the ER had no controller medication in the past year, despite evidence of persistent disease (Stempel, Roberts, & Stanford, 2004). The patient and family may be receptive to education at the time of ER visit because of the severity of the attack. The nurse should keep these facts in mind while providing discharge instructions and assessing barriers to care. The ER is not typically a place for maintenance medications to be prescribed, but the nurse can advocate for the patient by encouraging inclusion of controller medications in the discharge plan.

Discharge instructions include proper peak flow measuring and MDI technique, use of the written asthma action plan, and avoidance of the trigger that precipitated the current visit. If the patient is discharged with corticosteroids to keep on hand for future exacerbations, the nurse should review indications to take these as well. The importance of contacting the primary care provider or asthma specialist within 24 hours must be stressed. Patients who are followed up on within a few days of ER visits do better than patients who lack follow up. Patients who visit the ER are high risk for relapse and the nurse should refer them to asthma education programs (NHLBI/WHO, 2003).

THE HOSPITALIZED PERSON WITH ASTHMA

Criteria for Admission

Patients who do not respond to ER treatment after 1 to 2 hours should be monitored continuously. Other patients who require continuous monitoring include those with:

- persistent airflow limitation, peak flow < 30% predicted
- history of severe asthma or high risk of death
- prolonged symptoms prior to ER presentation

- inadequate access to medical care
- difficult home situation, including transportation to the hospital

Patients are hospitalized if asthma is severe or if posttreatment peak flow is < 40% predicted. Hospital care is a continuation of ER care with tapering of the beta$_2$-agonist. Systemic corticosteroids are continued because their use results in earlier discharge and fewer relapses (Smith, Iqbal, Elliott, & Rowe, 2003).

Nursing Implications

The nurse should recognize that hospital admission commonly is a result of the patient's nonadherence to the treatment plan. Hospitalization is a frightening experience, thus the patient may be open to education in this setting. The nurse should review the patient's understanding of the cause of the exacerbation, the purpose of treatment, the correct use of medications, and what actions to take when symptoms worsen. Hospitalized patients should also be referred to asthma education programs. The importance of prompt and regular follow-up should be stressed. If the patient's asthma is life threatening, or if the patient has experienced multiple hospitalizations because of asthma, the patient should be referred to an asthma specialist (NHLBI/WHO, 2003).

Nursing education positively impacts patient outcomes. Nursing education interventions coupled with support for overcoming social and healthcare access barriers significantly reduces repeat hospitalizations, missed work or school days, and healthcare costs (Castro, Zimmermann, Crocker, Bradley, Leven, & Schechtman, 2003).

SUMMARY

Signs and symptoms of acute asthma attacks must be recognized and treated promptly. Ideally, early treatment is initiated at home and based on a written action plan and consultation.

Those who do not respond completely to home treatment need referral to the ER. Principles of acute management in the ER include continuous pulse oximetry and peak flow monitoring, administration of oxygen, rapid-acting bronchodilators and systemic corticosteroids. Patients at risk for near-fatal asthma need to be identified, closely monitored, and given intense education and follow-up care. Goals of acute asthma education include recognizing the trigger that precipitated the episode, learning preventive strategies and proper use of peak flow and MDI devices, and reviewing medications. Nursing interventions have been shown to positively impact patient outcomes.

CASE STUDY

Michael, age 17, has moderate persistent asthma. He finds it difficult to take his daily controller medication because of his busy school and athletics schedule. He is on the football team this year. Michael recognizes that in the past, fall was his worst asthma season, but he believes that he has "outgrown" his asthma and admits that he has not used controller medication in more than a year. At presentation to the ER, Michael is unable to perform a peak flow maneuver. Spirometry indicates severe obstruction. He improves slightly after three albuterol treatments and is started on prednisone.

Michael's history reveals that he has used four canisters of albuterol in the past 6 months and has made several urgent care visits, which resulted in three courses of oral steroids. When asked if he usually has difficulty breathing, he states that he is not aware of difficulty until "it gets really bad."

Answer the following study questions, writing your responses on a separate sheet of paper. Compare your responses with the answers located at the end of the chapter.

1. What characteristics of near-fatal asthma are consistent with Michael's history?

2. What does Michael's inability to perform a peak flow maneuver suggest about the severity of his attack?

3. What factor helps explain Michael's poor response to the three albuterol treatments?

4. What are your priority education concerns for Michael?

Answers to Case Study

1. Michael has several characteristics of near-fatal asthma: poor perception of airway obstruction, several urgent care visits, lack of current controller medication, and overreliance on rescue medication.

2. Michael's inability to perform a peak flow maneuver is most likely because of severe obstruction. He has no primary care provider and may also not have received peak flow instruction.

3. Michael has been using excessive amounts of albuterol. Overuse of rapid-acting bronchodilators down regulates the receptor sites; which means there are fewer receptor sites available. The drug is less effective because it is activated by attaching to the sites. A priority in Michael's care is to reduce his reliance on albuterol.

4. Michael must be taught the importance of daily controller medication. He needs to be instructed in the use of a peak flow meter because his perception of airway obstruction is poor. He may need assistance finding a primary care provider, because he needs close monitoring. He should understand the importance of calling for an appointment within the next 24 hours. The nurse should also help Michael understand what trigger caused this visit and focus on avoidance of this trigger. He should also receive a written care plan with strategies for improving adherence, such as fitting medication times into his busy schedule.

EXAM QUESTIONS

CHAPTER 10
Questions 56-62

56. Symptoms of an acute asthma attack include

    a. inspiratory stridor.

    b. cough.

    c. rales.

    d. increased inspiratory to expiratory ratio.

57. An asthma attack is classified as "severe" when signs and symptoms include

    a. decreasing respiratory rate.

    b. lying in the supine position.

    c. speaking in words, not sentences.

    d. wheezing during expiration only.

58. Home management of an acute asthma attack includes prompt administration of

    a. albuterol.

    b. salmeterol.

    c. montelukast.

    d. ipratropium.

59. A characteristic of the person at high risk for death related to asthma includes

    a. current use of inhaled corticosteroids.

    b. infrequent use of beta$_2$-agonists.

    c. history of intubation.

    d. activity intolerance.

60. The goals of acute asthma care in the ER include

    a. review of all potential triggers.

    b. revision of the asthma action plan.

    c. enrollment in smoking cessation programs.

    d. identification of the current triggering event.

61. When providing education to the person with an acute asthma attack in the ER, the nurse should stress the importance of

    a. immediate follow-up within 24 hours.

    b. referral to a specialist.

    c. around-the-clock beta$_2$-agonists for 3 weeks.

    d. continuing the long-acting beta$_2$-agonist.

62. Severe attacks that result in hospital admission are usually the result of

    a. nonadherence to the treatment plan.

    b. emotional triggers.

    c. URIs.

    d. lack of regular primary care.

REFERENCES

Camargo, C., Spooner, C., & Rowe, R. (2003). *Continuous versus intermittent beta-agonists for acute asthma.* Retrieved, September 13, 2004, from Cochrane Database of Systematic Reviews.

Castro, M., Zimmermann, N., Crocker, S., Bradley, J., Leven, C., & Schechtman, K. (2003). Asthma intervention program prevents readmissions in high health care users. *American Journal of Critical Care Medicine, 168,* 1095-1099.

Corbridge. S. & Corbridge, T. (2004). Severe exacerbations of asthma. *Critical Care Nursing Quarterly, 27*(3), 207-228.

Gorelick, M., Stevens, M., Schultz, T., & Scribano, P. (2004). Difficulty in obtaining peak expiratory flow rates in children with acute asthma. *Pediatric Emergency Care, 20*(1), 22-26.

Kress, J., Noth, I., Gehlbach, B., Barman, N., Pohlman, A., Miller, A., et al. (2002). The utility of albuterol nebulized with heliox during acute asthma exacerbations. *American Journal of Critical Care Medicine, 165,* 1317-1321.

Magadle, R., Berar-Yanay, N., & Weiner, P. (2002). The risk of hospitalization and near-fatal and fatal asthma in relation to the perception of dyspnea. *Chest, 121*(2), 329-333.

Mitchell, I., Tough, S., Semple, L., Green, F., & Hessel, P. (2002). Near-fatal asthma: A population-based study of risk factors. *Chest, 121*(5), 1407-1413.

Moloney, E., O'Sullivan, S., Hogan, T., Poulter, L., & Burke, C. (2002). Airway dehydration: A therapeutic target in asthma? *Chest, 121*(6), 1806-1811.

National Asthma Education and Prevention Program. (1997). Expert panel report 2. *Guidelines for the diagnosis and management of asthma.* (NIH Publication No. 97-4051). Bethesda, MD: National Institutes of Health, National Heart, Lung, and Blood Institute. Available online at www.nhlbi.nih.gov/guidelines/asthma/index.pdf

National Asthma Education and Prevention Program. (2003). Expert Panel Report: *Guidelines for the diagnosis and management of asthma: Update on selected topics 2002.* (NIH Publication No. 02-5074). Bethesda, MD: National Institutes of Health, National Heart, Lung and Blood Institute. Available online at http://www.nhlbi.nih.gov/guidelines/asthma/index.html

National Heart, Lung, and Blood Institute/World Health Organization. (2003). *Global initiative for asthma: Global strategy for asthma management and prevention.* (NIH Publication No. 02-3659). Retrieved September 12, 2002, from http://www.ginasthma.com

Parameswaran, K., Belda, J., & Rowe, B. (2000). *The addition of intravenous aminophylline to beta2-agonists in adults with acute asthma.* Retrieved September 13, 2004, from Cochrane Database of Systematic Reviews.

Plotnick, L. & Ducharme, F. (2000). *Combined inhaled anticholinergics and beta$_2$-agonists for initial treatment of acute asthma in children.* Retrieved, September 13, 2004 from Cochrane Database of Systematic Reviews.

Rodrigo, G. & Rodrigo, C. (2002). The role of anticholinergics in acute asthma treatment: An evidenced-based evaluation. *Chest, 121*(6), 1977-1987.

Rowe, B., Spooner, C., Ducharme, F., Bretzlaff, J., & Bota, G. (2001). *Early emergency department treatment of acute asthma with systemic corticosteroids.* Retrieved September 13, 2004, from Cochrane Database of Systematic Reviews.

Silverman, R., Osborn, H., Runge, J., Gallagher, J., Chiang, W., Feldman, J., et al. (2002). IV magnesium sulfate in the treatment of acute severe asthma: A multicenter randomized controlled trial. *Chest, 122*(2), 489-497.

Smith, M., Iqbal, S., Elliott, T., & Rowe, B. (2003). *Corticosteroids for hospitalized children with acute asthma.* Retrieved September 13, 2004, from Cochrane Database of Systematic Reviews.

Stempel, D, Roberts, C., & Stanford, R. (2004). Treatment patterns in the months prior to and after asthma-related emergency department visit. *Chest, 126*(1), 75-80.

Travers, A., Jones, A., Kelly, K, Barker, S., Camargo, C., & Rowe, B. (2001). *Intravenous beta$_2$-agonists for acute asthma in the emergency department.* Retrieved September 13, 2004, from Cochrane Database of Systematic Reviews.

CHAPTER 11

EXERCISE-INDUCED ASTHMA

CHAPTER OBJECTIVE

Upon completion of this chapter, the reader will be able to identify signs and symptoms of exercise-induced asthma (EIA) and provide basic education to the patient and family regarding control of EIA and participation in sports.

LEARNING OBJECTIVES

After studying this chapter, the reader will be able to

1. define EIA.

2. state four symptoms associated with EIA.

3. recognize EIA symptoms as an indicator of poor asthma control.

4. identify three strategies for managing EIA.

5. recognize the benefit of regular exercise for most people with asthma.

6. state the nurse's role in referral and education.

INTRODUCTION

Sports and other physical activities, such as dancing or playing a musical instrument that requires respiratory effort such as a horn, are experiences that enrich life. A goal of asthma therapy is to encourage full participation in all activities, including sports. To help the patient achieve this goal, it is important for the nurse to understand EIA.

This chapter focuses on the pathophysiology, symptoms, prevalence, and treatment of EIA.

DEFINITION

EIA is an acute, self-limiting episode of bronchospasm caused by physical exertion. Exercise is one of the most common triggers of bronchospasm, affecting approximately 90% of people with asthma (Brooks, 2003) as well as 10% of healthy people (Sheth, 2003). Symptoms appear minutes into strenuous exercise, peak 5 to 10 minutes after stopping, and resolve 20 to 30 minutes later (National Asthma Education and Prevention Program [NAEPP], 1997). These symptoms differ from normal dyspnea caused by lack of fitness, which does not continue after the activity stops.

Most people with asthma experience some exercise-related symptoms. However, many adults, including those with asthma, are not meeting the current recommendations for physical exercise (Ford, Heath, Mannino, & Redd, 2003); therefore, exercise intolerance is probably under-reported in adults. Discussion of EIA usually focuses on children and young adults because adults fail to exercise and because children and young adults are most likely to be involved in sports.

PATHOPHYSIOLOGY OF EIA

Several theories have been tested regarding the pathophysiology of EIA. Research continues to explore precise mechanisms related to the pathophysiology of EIA. Two competing hypotheses currently have support in the literature. The thermal hypothesis maintains that during exercise airways cool as a result of rapid air exchange. Airway cooling is followed by rewarming; however, the airways of patients with asthma rewarm two times faster than airways of those without asthma. Rapid rewarming is thought to contribute to EIA symptoms (Cummiskey, 2001).

Another hypothesis—the osmotic hypothesis—suggests that EIA is caused by evaporation of water from the airway during exercise-related hyperventilation. Loss of water in the airway causes the liquid on the airway surface to become hyperosmolar. As water moves out of nearby cells, drying stimulates mast cell degranulation and contraction of airway smooth muscles (Sheth, 2003). Airway smooth muscles are less responsive to bronchodilator stimuli when cooled and become more responsive to bronchoconstrictor stimuli.

CONDITIONS THAT ENHANCE EIA

Certain conditions and types of exercise are more commonly associated with EIA. Sports that require sustained strenuous exercise, such as long-distance running, cycling, soccer, and cross-country skiing are commonly associated with EIA. Sports that require short bursts of activity, such as swimming, gymnastics, football, and baseball, are usually better tolerated. Exercising in cold, dry air places the person with asthma at greater risk than exercising in warm, humid environments (Cummiskey, 2001). Other factors capable of inducing EIA include high pollen levels and pollution (Sheth, 2003), especially sulfur dioxide and ozone. In fact, children participating in sports in polluted environments are also at risk for developing new onset asthma (McConnell et al., 2002).

SIGNS AND SYMPTOMS

Symptoms of EIA appear about 6 minutes into vigorous exercise. They are caused by bronchospasm and include shortness of breath, wheeze, cough, tight chest, and dyspnea (Cummiskey, 2001). These symptoms are variable among children. Some children experience primarily shortness of breath and tight chest, whereas others experience primarily cough or wheeze. Many children with asthma limit their physical activity to avoid respiratory discomfort and may not tell an adult that they have experienced symptoms. In assessing the child with asthma, the healthcare provider should be alert to a sedentary activity pattern as a possible indicator of exercise intolerance.

Episodes of breathlessness in children are frightening for adults. Parents and coaches may teach children to limit activity to avoid attacks. In sports, coaches may designate children with asthma to less active positions such as goalie. These practices result in children who are physically unfit and miss socialization opportunities. According to the guidelines developed by the National Asthma Education and Prevention Program (1997), physical activity and organized sports are essential parts of a child's life. Full participation should be encouraged.

DIAGNOSIS OF EIA

Interestingly, EIA may go undiagnosed or be undertreated (Sheth, 2003). Twenty per cent of healthy high school athletes in an inner-city middle school had abnormal pulmonary function tests during routine pre-sports screening tests (Brooks, 2003). On the other hand, EIA may be overdiagnosed in elite athletes. Unusually high rates of asthma are reported in

U.S. Olympic athletes, with rates ranging from 20% in summer games participants to 60% in winter games participants (Sheth, 2003). Some studies show that athletes with asthma win proportionately more medals than would be expected. The International Olympic Committee is currently investigating the effect of stimulant use on performance (Cummiskey, 2003). There may be overreporting among athletes because of the mistaken belief that rescue medication enhances performance.

A detailed history is important for accurate diagnosis (Sheth, 2003), but EIA can be difficult to assess for a number of reasons. Perception of symptoms is known to be poor. Parents as well as children often fail to recognize symptoms. Also, children may lack interest in physical activity, perceive that they are out of shape (Sheth, 2003), feel inadequate, or fear inability to continue playing (Sinha & David, 2003) if they report symptoms.

The nurse should refer a child or young adult who is suspected of having EIA for a complete physical examination. Symptoms and alterations in pulmonary functions tests can usually be demonstrated after having the child run in place for 10 minutes. Pulmonary function testing and exercise challenge testing are more reliable than history alone in confirming the diagnosis of EIA (Sinha & David, 2003).

EIA AS AN INDICATOR OF ASTHMA CONTROL

In most cases, activity intolerance is an indicator of poor asthma control (Brooks, 2003). Increased activity intolerance in patients with asthma can be used as a marker of asthma control. EIA symptoms are related to the degree of obstruction present in the airway before exercise (Sheth, 2003). In other words, the more obstruction present before exercise, the more severe the episode will be. EIA is also more severe during pollen season and following

upper respiratory infections, because these conditions cause increased airway inflammation.

Increased activity intolerance can be an indication that a person's asthma is becoming more severe, that exposure to environmental triggers is worsening inflammation, or that the medication plan is not being followed. As such, EIA can be thought of as an early warning sign that anti-inflammatory medication needs to be increased. It may be useful, particularly in children who are literal thinkers, to avoid classifying exercise as a trigger because a main concept of asthma education is to avoid triggers. People with asthma should not avoid exercise. Explaining exercise intolerance as an early warning sign should alert the child and family to take action to increase controller medication or seek professional help (Brooks, personal communication, July 11, 2004).

MANAGEMENT OF EIA

Pharmacotherapy

Short-acting inhaled beta$_2$-agonists taken 5 to 15 minutes before exercise effectively control symptoms in most patients. Short-acting beta$_2$-agonists are standard in most settings and include albuterol or pirbuterol (Brooks, 2003). The dose is 2 puffs (90 mcg/puff for albuterol; 200 mcg/puff for pirbuterol) via metered-dose inhaler (MDI) with spacer. Cromolyn sodium and nedocromil are similar acting nonsteroidal agents that are safe and inhibit symptoms in 70% to 87% of patients (Sheth, 2003); however, these drugs are not effective if given during or after activity. Nonsteroidals may be used as add-on therapy for individuals who do not have complete relief with beta$_2$-agonists alone. They are taken 30 minutes prior to activity.

Appropriate use of these medications requires consideration of behavioral issues. For example, use of beta$_2$-agonists requires planning, which is difficult for children, who are by nature spontaneous in their physical activity. The school-age child may also be unwilling to take medication in front of peers and may be anxious about managing EIA because of school policies that restrict them from carrying medication. Support from the school nurse may be sufficient in managing these issues, but if concerns persist, use of a long-acting beta$_2$-agonist may be considered.

Salmeterol, a long-acting bronchodilator (LAB) reduces symptoms and is effective over a period of 9 hours. An advantage of salmeterol for children with EIA is that it can be taken at home to avoid the need to medicate at school. The onset of action is 3 hours; therefore, salmeterol must be taken ahead of time (Brooks, 2003). Unfortunately, the effect of salmeterol lessens over time. After several months of treatment its effects are reduced. Formoterol is a newer LAB with a short onset of action—15 minutes—and it is effective for 12 hours. Some patients respond to leukotriene modifiers such as montelukast (Brooks, 2003).

The best therapy is prevention. Those with persistent forms of asthma receive the greatest EIA control from regular anti-inflammatory medication (Sheth, 2003). Inhaled corticosteroids (ICSs) are the primary treatment for EIA in persons with persistent asthma.

Athletes with asthma should avoid several drugs. Nonsteroidal anti-inflammatory drugs (NSAIDs) should not be used for pain relief because they may produce airway obstruction (Jenkins & Costello, 2004). In addition, over-the-counter epinephrine, sold as Primatine Mist or Bronchaid Mist, must be avoided because it increases acidosis and hypoxia. The athlete needs to be aware that oral or systemic glucocorticosteroids are banned in competition. A short-acting beta$_2$-agonist must be used sparingly to keep urine levels below 1,000 mg/mL. The usual controller medications, including ICSs are allowed in competition (Brooks, 2003).

Nonpharmacologic Measures

Nonpharmacologic measures must be included in the management of EIA. The young athlete should be counseled to select sports that are least likely to induce EIA (Cummiskey, 2001). Sports that take place in warm, humid environments and require short bursts of activity rather than endurance tends to be better tolerated. These include swimming, baseball, golf, diving, boxing, gymnastics, football, wrestling, and sprinting. Sports most likely to exacerbate EIA include long-distance running, cycling, cross country skiing, basketball, rugby, ice hockey, soccer, and ice skating (McConnell et al., 2001).

A slow warm-up with brief periods of intense activity and a slow cool down protect against bronchospasm (Brooks, 2003). Wearing a mask or using a muffler during cold weather helps lessen symptoms by providing extra humidity. Similarly, breathing through the nose decreases water loss. Children can be taught to use this technique for mild to moderately strenuous activity (Sinha & David, 2003). Controlled breathing and relaxation can be taught to help allay anxiety associated with bronchospasm (Brooks, 2003). There is also evidence that dietary fish oil supplements (Milgrom, 2004) and diets low in salt are protective against EIA (Sheth, 2003).

A primary goal of asthma management is full participation in all activities including sports. However, some occasions call for modification, such as when the pollen count or ozone level is high or when the athlete has a cold. Ozone is highest from 10 AM to 6 PM, so athletes may need to be counseled to play sports early in the morning, in the evening, or to avoid outdoor sports in high ozone areas (McConnell et al., 2002). Controller medication may need to be increased and activity may need to be limited.

BENEFITS OF EXERCISE

There are clearly many benefits of exercise for the person with asthma (Brooks, 2003). Exercise improves general health, emotional well-being, and physical appearance. It increases self-esteem, provides opportunities to socialize, enhances team-building skills, and may lead to a career or scholarship opportunities. On a physiologic level, improved physical fitness lessens the likelihood of EIA by reducing the ventilatory requirement for any activity (Milgrom, 2004). The fit athlete has an increased oxygen uptake and an ability to increase exercise intensity before reaching the threshold for EIA. In other words, the fit athlete experiences symptoms at a higher degree of physical activity than the unfit athlete. However, consistent evidence that physical training improves pulmonary functioning is lacking. The young athlete should not be misled to believe that asthma is overcome simply by training. The nurse should inform the athlete that good asthma management leads to the best athletic performance.

The nurse should also teach the person with asthma about the benefits of exercise and measures to avoid EIA. Misconceptions about exercise for the child with asthma need to be explored with parents, teachers, and coaches. The value of exercise as well as sound asthma management practices need to be communicated to all persons influencing the child's participation in sports (NAEPP, 1997).

SUMMARY

Most people with asthma experience some degree of exercise intolerance. Symptoms of bronchospasm typically occur shortly after beginning exercise. Endurance sports, exercising in cold or dry weather, pollution and high pollen counts are associated with EIA. EIA is often underdiagnosed and therefore undertreated, except in elite athletes who may mistakenly believe that rescue medication enhances performance. EIA in the person with existing asthma is an indicator of poor asthma control. Pharmacologic and nonpharmacologic measures to manage EIA were discussed. Most people with asthma benefit from exercise. The nurse should encourage patients to incorporate exercise into their asthma management plans.

CASE STUDY

Tim Smith, age 12, has moderate persistent asthma but is strongly motivated to play on the football team. Tim has come across campus to the nurse's clinic several times since the start of football season to use albuterol in the middle of the practice session. The coach is upset because Tim is missing half the practice sessions, and he is afraid that if the intensity of training is increased Tim may have a respiratory arrest. The coach is requesting a letter releasing him from all medical liability. What action should the nurse take?

Answer the following case study questions, writing your responses on a separate piece of paper. Compare your responses with the answers that are located at the end of the chapter.

1. What is the goal of care for Tim?

2. State four nursing assessment findings that determine Tim's management needs.

3. State three areas of concern that the school nurse must address with Tim's coach.

4. What asthma tool may help Tim make treatment decisions before exercise?

Answers to Case Study

1. The nurse should assist Tim in staying physically active. Football is a sport that is tolerated well by persons with asthma. To increase adherence, the nurse should include Tim in goal setting. Athletes are usually highly motivated to manage asthma if they understand the relationship of adherence to the medical plan and sports performance.

2. Exercise intolerance is commonly an indicator of poorly controlled asthma. The nurse should review Tim's adherence with daily controller medication and assess if Tim is taking rescue medication prior to play. If Tim is not following his asthma plan, what financial, social, and behavioral barriers exist? Assuming school policy permits students to carry their rescue inhaler, the nurse should assess Tim's maturity level for self-medication.

   The nurse should also assess what environmental factors might be triggering an asthma flare-up. Football season coincides with ragweed season—is Tim allergic to ragweed? Late summer is typically a hot time of the year. Ozone levels may be high. Is practice occurring in the late afternoon when ozone levels are highest?

3. The nurse must also consider the coach in the plan. The coach needs to understand that EIA is not a fatal condition, but is self-limiting. The coach must structure practice to permit a slow warm up and cool down. The nurse should also explain that Tim is receiving guidance to manage his asthma better and will use albuterol prior to practice, resulting in better control during practice. The coach should realize that if Tim has breathing difficulty on days when environmental triggers are problematic, he might have to miss practice.

4. The nurse should evaluate if use of a peak flow meter prior to practice would help guide decision making for Tim and the coach.

EXAM QUESTIONS

CHAPTER 11
Questions 63-68

63. EIA can best be described as an abnormal response of the airways to

   a. excessive humidification.

   b. rapid breathing.

   c. lactic acid produced during exercise.

   d. water loss and altered temperature.

64. Symptoms of EIA occur how soon after beginning a physical activity?

   a. 2 minutes

   b. 6 minutes

   c. 10 to 15 minutes

   d. 20 to 30 minutes

65. Symptoms of EIA include:

   a. tachycardia.

   b. excessive sweating.

   c. tight chest.

   d. runny nose.

66. Persons who are least likely to experience EIA include

   a. Olympic swimmers.

   b. healthy high school athletes.

   c. those with asthma who are using controller medication.

   d. those with asthma who are using controller medication and perform a 10 minute slow warm-up before exercise.

67. A high school athlete takes Primatene Mist® before playing football. The nurse should advise the student that Primatene Mist® will

   a. decrease the available oxygen to his body.

   b. open the airway as well as albuterol.

   c. have a rebound effect, causing increased airway narrowing.

   d. have a longer onset of action than albuterol.

68. The school nurse should advise that the athlete with asthma

   a. avoid participating in all endurance sports.

   b. be allowed to carry a rescue inhaler for mid-game dosing.

   c. avoid outdoor sports on high ozone days.

   d. do a quick warm-up and cool down.

REFERENCES

Brooks, E. & Hayden, M.L. (2003). Exercise-induced asthma. *Nursing Clinics of North America, 38*(4), 689-69.

Cummiskey, J. (2001). Exercise-induced asthma: An overview. *American Journal of Medical Science, 322*(4), 200-2003.

Ford, E., Heath, G., Mannino, D., & Redd, S. (2003). Leisure-time physical activity patterns among US adults with asthma. *Chest, 124*(2), 432-437.

Jenkins, C., Costello, J., & Hodge, L. (2004). Systematic review of prevalence of aspirin induced asthma and its implications for clinical practice. *British Medical Journal, 328*(7437), 434-449.

McConnell, R., Berhane, K., Gilliand, F., London, S., Islam, T., Gauderman, T., et al. (2002). Asthma in exercising children exposed to ozone: A cohort study. *The Lancet, 359,* 386-391.

Milgrom, H. (2004). Exercise-induced asthma: Wise ways to exercise. *Current Opinion in Clinical Immunology, 4*(3), 147-153.

National Asthma Education and Prevention Program. (1997). Expert panel report 2. *Guidelines for the diagnosis and management of asthma.* (NIH Publication No. 97-4051). Bethesda, MD: National Institutes of Health, National Heart, Lung, and Blood Institute. Available online at www.nhlbi.nih.gov/guidelines/asthma/index.pdf

National Heart, Lung, and Blood Institute/World Health Organization. (2003). *Global initiative for asthma:* Global strategies for asthma management and prevention. (NIH Publication No. 02-3659). Retrieved November 12, 2003, from http://www.ginasthma.com

Sheth, K. (2003). Activity-induced asthma. *Pediatric Clinics of North America, 50*(3). Retrieved August 19, 2004, from http://home.mdconsult.com

Sinha, T. & David, A. (2003). Recognition and management of exercise-induced bronchospasm. *American Family Physician, 67*(4), 769–774.

CHAPTER 12

ALLERGY AND ASTHMA-RELATED CONDITIONS

CHAPTER OBJECTIVE

Upon completion of this chapter, the reader will be able to recognize the impact of co-morbid diseases such as atopic dermatitis, allergic rhinitis, sinusitis, and gastroesophageal reflux on optimal asthma control.

LEARNING OBJECTIVES

After studying this chapter, the reader will be able to

1. identify the atopic triad.

2. state five pathologic similarities between atopic dermatitis, allergic rhinitis and asthma.

3. identify two commonalities in the management of atopic dermatitis, allergic rhinitis, and asthma.

4. state what is meant by the term "united airway disease."

5. recognize the impact of allergic rhinitis on quality of life, health costs, and disease progression.

6. recognize five common clinical findings in a person with allergic rhinitis.

7. identify the impact of sinusitis on asthma control.

8. recognize the interrelationship of asthma and gastroesophageal reflux (GER) symptoms and identify three strategies to control GER.

9. identify the importance of educating the person with allergy or GER about how to control symptoms.

OVERVIEW

Most people with asthma suffer from comorbid conditions. Allergic rhinitis is the most common condition seen in patients with asthma. Sinusitis, atopic dermatitis, and GER commonly complicate asthma management. Allergic rhinitis, in particular, has a major impact on asthma. A large number of evidenced-based studies now indisputably link allergic rhinitis to asthma. Because of this, the World Health Organization formed a work group to suggest strategies for the development of treatment guidelines for allergic rhinitis based on the scientific data from these studies (Bosquet, van Cauwenberge, & Khaltaev, 2001). This state-of-the-art document, commonly referred to as the ARIA report (Allergic Rhinitis and its Impact on Asthma), is the foundation of much of the discussion in this chapter.

Topics reviewed in this chapter include common pathologic features of the allergic comorbidities, interaction of comorbid conditions with asthma, and treatment measures for these diseases. The nurse should actively suspect any of these comorbid conditions in patients with asthma and appreciate the importance of controlling these conditions for optimal asthma control.

THE ATOPIC TRIAD

Atopic dermatitis, allergic rhinitis, and asthma share many pathologic features and commonly occur in the same individuals. Because of their commonalities, these conditions have been labeled as the "atopic triad." Atopic dermatitis often progresses to allergic rhinitis and then to asthma—the so-called "allergic march" (Helm, 2004). This concept of progression is controversial because there is evidence that genetic or environmental "lung factors" may predetermine whether a person will develop asthma, regardless of the presence of atopic dermatitis (Casale & Dykewicz, 2004). However, both atopic dermatitis and allergic rhinitis are risk factors for asthma and, like asthma, their prevalence is increasing in the developed world. There is current interest in early identification and treatment of atopic dermatitis and allergic rhinitis to determine potential impact of early treatment on incidence and severity of asthma.

Atopic Dermatitis

The lifetime prevalence of atopic dermatitis is 10% to 20% in children and 1% to 3% in adults. Atopic dermatitis prevalence has increased two to three times in industrialized countries in the last 30 years. The hygiene hypothesis (the lack of early life exposures to infectious illness, which fails to stimulate the development of protective immunoglobins) is thought to explain this increase. Similar to asthma, there is a high familial occurrence of atopic dermatitis, and the interplay of genetics and environmental triggers contribute to the expression of this skin disorder.

Pathophysiology

Exposure to cow's milks, egg protein, and other food allergens early in infancy can lead to atopic dermatitis (Helm, 2004). Like asthma, atopic dermatitis is a chronic inflammatory disease. In atopic dermatitis the skin reacts excessively (hyperreactivity) to environmental triggers that are not irritants to most people. This parallels the hyperreactivity of asthmatic airways to innocuous stimuli.

In infants, atopic dermatitis usually presents as a dry, pruritic rash (eczema) of the face. In the young child, the rash is more prominent on the extensor surfaces of the extremities. Atopic dermatitis has typically been considered a childhood disease. Although it commonly improves by age 6, it can persist or start in adulthood. The main feature in adults is an eczematous rash in the flexural creases of the extremities (Leung, Boguniewicz, Howell, Nomura, & Hamid, 2004).

The atopic dermatitis rash is characteristically erythematous with papulovesicular lesions that weep and crust. Itching is intense and leads to scratching, which in turn can cause secondary bacterial infection. Over time, the weeping lesions progress to reddened, scaling patches. Eventually, chronic lichenified (thickened, hardened) skin patches form (Helm, 2004). Lichenified skin is the result of chronic inflammation and, like thickened basement membranes in asthmatic airways, is a form of remodeling. Skin that is unaffected by lesions in atopic dermatitis is not normal because it contains more Th2 (inflammatory mediators) cells than normal, it is very dry, and it is more easily irritated than normal skin.

As in asthma, the immunologic and inflammatory pathways in atopic dermatitis are complex. Atopic dermatitis appears to be the manifestation in the skin of a systemic disorder that also gives rise to allergic rhinitis and asthma. Each of these diseases is characterized by increased serum immunoglobulin (Ig) E levels and eosinophilia. Atopic dermatitis is often the first step in the march to allergic rhinitis and asthma (Leung et al., 2004).

Unlike asthma, food allergy commonly triggers the cycle of itching, scratching, and skin flaring in atopic dermatitis. After age 3, children tend to outgrow food allergy but become sensitized to inhalant allergens. Like asthma, viruses and inhaled allergens can exacerbate skin lesions, and the degree of sensitization to allergens is associated with the severity of atopic dermatitis.

Management

Treatment of atopic dermatitis is similar to asthma treatment in many respects. The goal of treatment is to stop the itch-scratch cycle. The first-line treatment includes administration of antihistamines, lubrication of the skin, and trigger avoidance. The mainstay of pharmacologic management for the past 40 years has been anti-inflammatory treatment with topical corticosteroids. However, two new immunomodulating agents, tacrolimus and pimecrolimus are now available (Pascual & Fleischer, 2004). They are supplied as topical creams. Both suppress inflammation by inhibiting T cell activation. These agents do not cause thinning of the skin and can be used for months or years on all skin areas, including the face. Both agents are safe in adults and children older than age 2, but tacrolimus can cause temporary burning and itching. Tacrolimus is equivalent in action to mid-potency topical corticosteroids and is indicated for moderate to severe atopic dermatitis. Pimecrolimus is less potent and is indicated for mild to moderate atopic dermatitis.

In February of 2005, the Pediatric Food and Drug Advisory Committee recommended labeling changes for tacrolimus and pimecrolimus because of a potential cancer risk. The warning is based on animal studies and a limited number of human case reports. It will take years to determine the actual cancer risk in humans. In the meantime, use of these drugs will be limited to second-line therapy for patients who have not responded to other therapies. Because the effect of these drugs on the developing immune system is not known, they are not recommended in children younger than age 2. Use in older patients should be limited to a short course of therapy. Also, persons with compromised immune systems should not use tacrolimus or pimecrolimus (U.S. Food and Drug Administration, 2005).

Combination therapy with tacrolimus and topical corticosteroids appears to provide a synergistic effect with diminished adverse effects from either drug. More studies are needed to confirm these findings. Disease flares do fluctuate over time. The immunomodulating agents may not be sufficient to control symptoms from time to time. In such cases, topical corticosteroids need to be added to the treatment plan. Secondary infected eczematous lesions require antibiotics.

Specific skin care recommendations for atopic dermatitis include avoidance of rough fabrics and fragranced soaps or avoiding soap entirely. Bathing in tepid water, rather than hot water, is recommended because heat stimulates the release of histamine, which causes itching. A mild hydrating agent such as Eucerin® (cream or lotion) is applied after bathing. Best results are obtained if the cream or lotion is applied within 3 minutes of bathing in order to trap water in the dry skin. A 1% hydrocortisone cream can be added to Eucerin.®

Topical corticosteroids can cause thinning of the skin. Caution should be used when applying them on infants or the face. Topical corticosteroids should only be used intermittently to control acute exacerbations because of the risk of skin atrophy and systemic absorption.

Breast-feeding is a preventive measure in atopic dermatitis. Children who were exclusively breast-fed for 4 months or more have significantly less atopic dermatitis than infants receiving partial breast feeding. This protective effect was seen regardless of the presence of asthma or allergy in either parent (Helm, 2004).

Allergic Rhinitis

It has been recognized for over 100 years that there is a relationship between asthma and allergic rhinitis. Traditionally, upper airway disease (allergic rhinitis) and lower airway disease (asthma) were treated by different specialists and were therefore viewed as two distinct diseases. Research strategies lacked a combined approach. However, mounting evidence that these diseases are related has led to research focusing on the relationship of allergic rhinitis and asthma. It is now recognized that disease in the upper airway influences disease in the lower airway and vice versa and that many common pathologic features are shared in allergic rhinitis and asthma (Braunstahl & Hellings, 2003). This insight has led the World Asthma Organization to propose the term "united airway disease."

The intent of the "united airway" concept is to focus healthcare providers' awareness that the upper and lower airways function as one airway and to suspect a comorbid disease if either disease is present (Murray & Rusznak, 2003). Asthma should be assessed for in all persons with allergic rhinitis and allergic rhinitis assessed in all persons with asthma. Treatment for either should consider the potential effect on co-existing disease (Casale & Dykewicz, 2004).

Epidemiology

In recent years, the incidence of allergic rhinitis has increased 10% to 50% in developed countries. Reasons for this increase are thought to be changes in lifestyle; increased exposure to allergens, pollution, and smoke; decrease in protective dietary nutrient intake; decrease in infection, and increased stress (Bosquet et al. 2001).

Allergic rhinitis is a serious problem because it negatively affects quality of life, work and school productivity, and health costs. Increasing evidence makes it clear that people with allergic rhinitis are bothered by sleep disorders, emotional problems, and impairment in activities and social functioning. Physical and mental functioning is impaired by loss of vitality and perception of suboptimal general health (Bosquet et al., 2001). Children may have impaired school performance due to malaise associated with allergic rhinitis and loss of sleep.

Approximately 20% of persons of all ages from all over the world have allergic rhinitis (Taramarcaz & Gibson, 2003). Up to 40% of those with allergic rhinitis have asthma, and 80% to 99% of people with asthma have nasal symptoms (Pawankar, 2004; Casale & Dykewicz, 2004).

People with allergic rhinitis are three times as likely to develop asthma than people without allergic rhinitis. Infants who develop allergic rhinitis are twice as likely to develop asthma than those children who develop rhinitis after the first year of life (Pawankar, 2004). As in asthma, living on a farm, exposure to animals, and a large family reduce the risk of developing allergic rhinitis (Braunstahl & Hellings, 2003; Boulay & Boulet, 2003).

Allergic rhinitis is one of the top ten reasons for clinic visits. Associated health costs are high. Direct medical costs for allergic rhinitis are estimated at $1.2 billion annually. This figure does not account for over-the-counter medication or indirect costs such as work and school absenteeism. People who have both allergic rhinitis and asthma pay an estimated 46% more annually for medications than those with asthma alone (Casale & Dykewicz, 2004).

Pathophysiology

Allergic rhinitis is a symptomatic disorder of the nose caused by IgE mediated inflammation that occurs after nasal membranes are exposed to allergens. The pathophysiology of allergic rhinitis is similar to asthma. Both are chronic immunologic diseases that are inflammatory in nature, both have a strong genetic basis, and both have the same allergens and irritants triggers. With respect to triggers, outdoor allergens are more related to allergic rhinitis, wheras indoor allergens are more related to asthma (Boulay & Boulet, 2003).

The nose, trachea, and bronchi are all lined with columnar epithelium, which is indistinguishable in the laboratory. Airway epithelium plays a central role in progression of disease in both asthma and allergic rhinitis by releasing inflammatory mediators (Murray & Rusnack, 2003). Many of the mediators that stimulate inflammation in asthma also produce inflammation in allergic rhinitis, and eosinophils are found in both lower airway and upper airway tissue. Like asthma, allergic rhinitis begins with allergen sensitization via activated Th2 helper cells. After an inhaled allergen settles in the nose, Th2 sensitization results in production of allergen-specific IgE, which, in turn, activates the mast cell to set the inflammatory cascade in motion (Casale & Dykewicz, 2004).

Like asthma, allergic rhinitis has an early and late phase response. Rhinorrhea (runny nose), sneezing, itching, and obstruction occur within minutes of allergen exposure. Nasal histamine release is responsible for sneezing and itching. Plasma leakage from the rich nasal vasculature causes nasal congestion in the early phase. Changes in blood flow through the nasal mucosa can rapidly expand or shrink the size of the nasal cavities and is a key feature in obstruction of the nasal passages (Bosquet et al., 2001). However, vasomotor and glandular stimulation, as opposed to airway smooth muscle in asthma, contribute to nasal obstruction in the early phase.

After initial allergen exposure, inflammatory mediators are recruited into nasal tissue. These mediators continue to recruit inflammatory mediators in a self-sustaining process identical to the process in the lower airways in asthma. Over the next 4 to 8 hours, a more prolonged late phase response results in nasal congestion and increased sensitivity to inhaled allergens or irritants. Nasal congestion in allergic rhinitis is analogous to bronchoconstriction in asthma (Casale & Dykewicz, 2004).

To further establish the allergic rhinitis–asthma link, it has been noted that those with allergic rhinitis have hyperresponsive lower airways, even if they do not have asthma. Inhalation of allergens into the nose further increases this lower airway hyperresponsiveness (Pawankar, 2004). This particular link is the focus of intense research.

It is known that precursors of inflammatory mediators for both asthma and allergic rhinitis are located in the bone marrow. There is some evidence for crosstalk between the upper and lower airways via the blood stream and bone marrow. If this is indeed the case, future therapy may be aimed at sys-

temic approaches rather than the current inhaled approaches (Braunstahl & Hellings, 2003).

Allergic rhinitis has some differences from asthma. The function of the nose is different from the lower airway. The nose acts as a filter to reduce the exposure of allergens and irritants to the lower airway. As noted above, nasal tissue is extremely vascular. This rich microvasculature heats, warms, and regulates flow of inspired air. Nasal capillaries are fenestrated, or windowed, which allows plasma to flow easily, creating exudate for copious secretions. Inflammation leads to excessive secretion, resulting in nasal congestion and rhinorrhea—the characteristic symptoms of allergic rhinitis. Unlike asthma, little epithelium is shed in the nose and remodeling is less pronounced (Casale & Dykewicz, 2004).

Risk Factors for the Development of Allergic Rhinitis

A positive family history of allergy, especially history of allergic rhinitis, is the greatest risk factor for development of allergic rhinitis. Other risk factors include early introduction of solid foods in infancy, heavy smoking by the mother in the first year of life, and pollen allergy (Bosquet et al., 2001).

Theories for the Allergic Rhinitis – Asthma Link

The exact cause of the interaction between asthma and allergic rhinitis is not well understood, but several hypotheses have been proposed. One hypothesis suggests that mouth breathing due to nasal congestion bypasses the warming and filtering effect of the nose. The lower airway is then directly exposed to cold, dry air with an increased allergen or irritant load. Support for this hypothesis is seen in exercise-induced asthma in athletes due to mouth breathing of cold, dry air. Laboratory studies have also documented decreases in pulmonary function when cold air is introduced into the lower airways (Boulay & Boulet, 2003).

A second hypothesis suggests that nasal inflammatory mediators may be drained into the lower airway by a postnasal drip mechanism (Koh & Kim,

2003). There is no scientific evidence to support this concept, but there is some indirect evidence that inflammatory mediators may reach the lung by a systemic route. This evidence is supported by the observation that nasal challenge with allergens increases the number of inflammatory mediators found in the bronchial mucosa.

It is known that the upper and lower airways share a common neural pathway. An additional hypothesis, based on airway response to histamine, suggests that inflammation in the nose stimulates inflammation in the lower airway by a neural reflex under central nervous system control. Histamine causes bronchoconstriction and is commonly used in the laboratory to measure hyperresponsiveness in the lung. When histamine is introduced in the nose, pulmonary function in the lower airway significantly declines. The reverse is also true—when the lower airway is challenged with histamine, increased nasal airflow resistance is observed.

The asthma–allergic rhinitis link is extremely complex and probably involves several pathways. Needless to say, more research is needed to determine the exact cause.

Triggers for Allergic Rhinitis

The triggers for allergic rhinitis are identical to asthma triggers. They include smoking, GER, and drugs such as aspirin and nonsteroidal anti-inflammatory drugs. People with perennial nasal symptoms are usually allergic to house dust mites, whereas people with seasonal allergy are usually sensitized to pollen. Tree pollen predominates in the spring, grass in the late spring and summer, and weed in late summer and fall. The first pollen of the season "primes" the nose and after priming, it takes less pollen to produce symptoms. Ozone levels generally increase during pollen season. The nose absorbs up to 40% of inhaled ozone and ozone increases the late phase response to allergens (Bosquet et al. 2001).

People with allergic rhinitis commonly develop nasal hyperreactivity and experience symptoms after exposure to irritants such as cold air, smoke, and strong odors. As with asthma, primary therapy is trigger avoidance. (See chapter 6 for trigger avoidance strategies.)

Clinical Findings

Initial symptoms of allergic rhinitis include sneezing, nasal pruritis, and clear rhinorrhea. Nasal congestion develops later. Patients with dust mite sensitivity usually complain of increased stuffiness early in the morning. Obstruction may be severe enough to interrupt sleep. Itching may also involve the eyes, ears, and throat. Children commonly relieve an itchy nose by pressing the palm of the hand upward against the nose in an "allergic salute." Constant rubbing can lead to a transverse crease across the lower third of the nose. When the nose is obstructed the person becomes a mouth breather and snoring becomes problematic during sleep.

The nasolacrimal duct drains into the nose and nasal obstruction impedes drainage, causing the vasculature under the eyes to become congested and producing the dark circles or "allergic shiners" commonly seen in people with allergic rhinitis. Allergic conjunctivitis is also commonly seen in people with allergic rhinitis. Severe nasal obstruction involves the sinuses, causes effusion in the middle ear that may affect hearing, and leads to loss of the senses of taste and smell.

Physical examination reveals swollen nasal turbinates, pale or sometimes purplish mucosa, watery discharge, and increased vascularity.

Classifications

Allergic rhinitis has traditionally been classified as seasonal, perennial, or occupational. Perennial allergic rhinitis is usually caused by indoor allergens. Seasonal allergic rhinitis is usually caused by outdoor allergens.

The recent ARIA initiative of the World Health Organization proposed a new classification

(Bousquet et al., 2001) mainly because it has become increasingly difficult to discriminate between seasonal and perennial nasal symptoms. Some seasonal allergens cause perennial symptoms whereas some perennial allergens cause symptoms only during certain times of the year. To further complicate the issue, most patients are sensitized to multiple allergens, creating confusion when identifying indoor or outdoor allergens as the culprits.

The new classification system is designed to simplify the description of allergic rhinitis. The basis of the new system is severity of symptoms and their impact on quality of life. The allergic rhinitis classification is identical to the classification used to describe asthma: intermittent, mild persistent, moderate persistent, or severe persistent. Intermittent allergic rhinitis means that symptoms are present less than 4 days per week or for less than 4 weeks. Mild means that sleep and activities are not affected (Bosquet et al. 2001). Because this classification involves new terminology, older terms will be used when referencing work based on the traditional classification of allergic rhinitis.

Management

Management of allergic rhinitis has received increased interest lately as a result of studies that indicate that treatment early in the course of the disease may prevent the occurrence of asthma, or at least decrease its severity (Bousquet et al., 2001) and prevent sensitization to new allergens (Fuhlbrigge & Adams, 2003). In fact, control of allergic rhinitis in people with mild asthma may reduce symptoms to such an extent that controller medication is not needed (Koh & Kim, 2003). People with asthma who are treated for allergic rhinitis experience about half as many emergency room visits and hospitalizations as people with asthma who do not receive allergic rhinitis treatment (Crystal-Peters, Neslusan, Crown, & Torres, 2002).

Management of allergic rhinitis is similar to asthma and includes trigger avoidance (see chapter 6), similar pharmacotherapy; and immunotherapy.

Pharmacotherapy

Symptoms of allergic rhinitis are caused by several different pathological mechanisms. No single class of drug is effective in controlling all symptoms. Several classes of medication are needed to manage allergic rhinitis: corticosteroids, antihistamines, decongestants, leukotriene modifiers, and the cromones. Drug choices in relation to classification of allergic rhinitis is listed in Table 12-1.

Routes of Administration

Routes of administration are intranasal or oral. There are advantages and disadvantages to each route. Generally, the intranasal route is preferred because high drug doses can be directly delivered to the target organ and systemic effects are avoided. Absorption is better and drugs have a quicker onset of action with intranasal administration.

Problems with the intranasal route include need for multiple dosing throughout the day and variable distribution throughout the nose. Some patients can be managed with once daily intranasal dosing but many require twice daily dosing. Approximately 50% of the medication administered by nasal sprays reaches the mucous membrane and very little probably reaches the sinuses. Another issue with nasal administration is that benzalkonium chloride is commonly used as a preservative in nasal sprays. This agent may act as an irritant, especially in people who have developed hyperresponsiveness to irritants. This effect tends to diminish over time as corticosteroids are administered (Bosquet et al., 2001).

Patients sometimes complain that the nasal spray "runs out of the nose." This is a sign of total nasal obstruction. Intranasal medication cannot be administered when nasal cavities are completely obstructed. Short-course oral steroids or decongestants are needed to relieve the obstruction and allow continuation of intranasal therapy. Patients also need instruction in proper administration of intranasal medication. The nose must be cleaned of secretions, the head must be tilted slightly forward, and the

TABLE 12-1: PHARMACOLOGIC MANAGEMENT OF ALLERGIC RHINITIS	
Severity of Allergic Rhinitis	**Treatment** (not in order of preference)
Mild intermittent	• Oral or intranasal H1-antihistamines • Intranasal decongestants (for < 10 days and not > 2 times/month • Oral decongestants (not usually recommended in children)
Moderate/severe intermittent	• Oral or intranasal H1-antihistamines • Oral H1-antihistamines and decongestants • Intranasal corticosteroids • Cromolyn or nedocromil
Mild persistent	• Oral or intranasal H1-antihistamines • Oral H1-antihistamines and decongestants • Intranasal corticosteroids with stepwise dosing approach as symptoms lessen or increase • Cromolyn or nedocromil
Moderate persistent	• Intranasal corticosteroids as first line, stepwise dosing • Short course oral corticosteroids if nose is blocked OR Intranasal decongestants for no more than 10 days • Oral H1-antihistamines for itching, sneezing, rhinorrhea • Ipratroprium chloride if major symptom is rhinorrhea • Oral H1-antihistamines and decongestants

Note. From Bosquet, J., van Cauwenberge, P., & Khaltaev, N. (2001). Allergic rhinitis and its impact on asthma (ARIA) in collaboration with the World Health Organization (WHO). *Journal of Allergy and Clinical Immunology, 108*, (Suppl), S147–S336. Reprinted with permission of Elsevier.

spray must be directed away from the nasal septum. Adherence to therapy is usually greater with oral medication, but education about the benefits of intranasal medication may increase adherence.

Antihistamines

Histamine acts mainly via H1 receptors. It causes the itching, sneezing, and watery rhinorrhea that is characteristic of allergic rhinitis. H1 antihistamines can control these symptoms. First generation antihistamines (such as diphenhydramine and chlorpheniramine) are very sedating and are associated with other central nervous system effects such as depression. For these reasons, they are not first-line choices for management of allergic rhinitis. Second generation H1 antihistamines are more potent, have a longer duration of action, and have minimal sedative effects. Not all antihistamines have similar effects. A person who does not respond to one antihistamine may respond to another. H1 antihistamines also act on non-nasal symptoms, such as allergic conjunctivitis, which is often present in patients with allergic rhini-

tis. Patients commonly report using antihistamines on an "as-needed" basis; however, long-term treatment is more effective than "as-needed" dosing. Furthermore, long-term treatment may improve lower airway symptoms in children.

Most of the new antihistamines have a rapid onset of action (1 to 2 hours) and effects last up to 24 hours. Drug interactions are common because some antihistamines are metabolized in the liver's cytochrome P450 system.

Antihistamines are usually oral medications but two intranasal preparations are available: azelastine (effective in children) and levocabastine. Azelastine is currently available on the market. At the time of this printing, intranasal levocabastine, which is being used successfully in Europe, is expected to become available in the United States in the near future.

Intranasal antihistamine preparations are advantageous because the drug can be delivered directly to the nose. Symptom relief occurs within 15 minutes. When these drugs are used twice per day, symptoms can even be prevented.

Corticosteroids

Early attempts to use intranasal corticosteroids (INSs) failed because they were either ineffective or caused systemic side effects. The situation changed when beclomethasone and later fluticasone and budesonide were introduced. INSs are the most potent medications for the treatment of allergic rhinitis and are the first line of therapy for people with moderate or severe symptoms. They are more effective when given before the onset of seasonal symptoms and when continued on a daily basis.

INSs are anti-inflammatory agents. They are effective in reducing nasal obstruction because such obstruction is caused by inflammation. Onset of action is slow (less than 12 hours) and maximal efficacy is not seen for days or weeks. Once daily dosing is usually adequate unless symptoms are severe, in which case dosing is increased to twice daily.

INSs are safe and have a minimal risk of side effects. They can be used long term without risk of nasal tissue atrophy. Rarely, some people may experience mild nosebleed and prolonged use can cause perforation of the nasal septum. Risk of perforation is reduced when the spray is aimed away from the septum. The newer INSs have no effect on the hypothalamic-pituitary axis (Bosquet et al., 2001).

Nonsteroidal Anti-inflammatory Agents

Cromolyn sodium and nedocromil are nonsteroidal medications with anti-inflammatory properties. The exact mode of action is not well understood, but the nonsteroidal agents appear to stabilize the mast cell. They are less potent than INSs and antihistamines but have an excellent safety record. Cromolyn has the disadvantage of four daily doses, so adherence to therapy is commonly poor. Nedocromil is effective when given twice daily. The nonsteroidal anti-inflammatory agents are rarely used in adults because other classes of drugs are more effective. Because of their excellent safety record, use is limited to children and pregnant women.

Leukotriene Modifiers

There is now supporting evidence for the role of leukotriene modifiers in seasonal allergic rhinitis. Recent data support that they have a role in the treatment of aspirin sensitive allergic rhinitis (Bosquet et al, 2001).

Decongestants

Decongestants act on the nasal vasculature to promote constriction. Examples are phenylephrine, ephedrine, pseudoephedrine, and phenylpropanolamine. They are administered orally or intranasally. In the short term, intranasal preparations are very effective in relieving nasal obstruction, usually within 10 minutes. Decongestants, however, have no effect on allergy symptoms (itching, sneezing, rhinorrhea). If used for longer than 10 days, intranasal decongestants become less effective and cause rebound congestion with the chronic swelling of "rhinitis medicamentosa." The decongestant must be stopped. Further treatment is controversial, but fluticasone has shown effect on rebound congestion.

Side effects of intranasal decongestants include burning, stinging, nasal dryness, or even septal perforation with prolonged use. Systemic side effects are uncommon but can include irritability, dizziness, headache, tremor, and insomnia.

Intranasal decongestants are useful as a short (3 day) course. They relieve nasal blockage and open the nasal passages to allow for deposition of antihistamine or steroid preparations. Patients tend to rely on medications that yield immediate relief. The importance of clearly explaining the need to limit decongestants to no more than a 3-day course cannot be overstated.

Oral decongestant preparations can be used either short or long term. Their effects are weaker than with the intranasal preparations but oral preparations have the advantage of no rebound congestion. Oral decongestants act within 30 minutes. Effects last up to 6 hours, or 24 hours with sustained-release formulations.

Decongestants have a narrow therapeutic range and should be used with caution in infants and during pregnancy. They should be avoided in older adults and in patients with cardiovascular disease. Over-the-counter preparations that combine decongestants with antihistamines should be avoided because the antihistamine is short acting and the stimulant effect of the decongestant does not counteract the sedating effect of the antihistamine.

Anticholinergics

The topical anticholinergic ipratropium bromide effectively blocks mucus secretion when administered three to six times daily. It is effective only on rhinorrhea. Ipratropium has a rapid onset with a duration of action of 3 hours. Tolerance does not develop. It is especially effective when combined with an INS. It is safe and causes minor side effects, including nasal dryness, irritation, burning, stuffy nose, dry mouth, and headache. Other drugs are preferred for first-line treatment, but ipratropium should be considered when rhinorrhea is the main symptom.

Immunotherapy

Immunotherapy is the administration of gradually increasing amounts of specific allergen vaccine to a person with allergen sensitivity in order to lessen symptoms when the person is exposed to that specific allergen. Immunotherapy is the only treatment that can alter the course of IgE mediated disease. It has been shown to significantly reduce the risk of asthma if started early in the course of disease.

Immunotherapy is 45% effective in reducing seasonal and perennial allergic rhinitis symptoms and in reducing the need for drugs (Bosquet et al., 2001). Effects last for about 3 years. This effect is greater than the effect of most drugs. It is indicated for those patients in need of constant treatment and is more effective if instituted early, before symptoms become severe. It is more effective in children

and young adults than later in life. There are currently no data to support treatment in infants or young children. Immunotherapy is generally started after age 5.

Immunotherapy has traditionally been administered subcutaneously, but local nasal and sublingual preparations are being studied in Europe. Dosages via these routes must be much higher than the subcutaneous route (Bosquet et al., 2001). Findings on the efficacy of nasal and sublingual immunotherapy are mixed, but these routes do not appear to be as effective as the subcutaneous route.

Immunotherapy requires administration by a specialist in a setting where anaphylaxis can be managed. The risk of anaphylaxis is lower in people with only allergic rhinitis than in people with asthma. Treatment is expensive and prolonged. Patients must also be receptive to the requirements of administering this therapy.

Immunotherapy is indicated for patients with allergic rhinitis, allergic conjunctivitis or asthma caused by pollen, house dust mite, or cat allergen; patients who cannot avoid triggers; patients whose medication does not adequately control symptoms; patients with undesirable side effects; and patients who do not want long term medication therapy.

SINUSITIS

Sinusitis is bacterial infection of the paranasal sinuses. The sinuses are air-filled cavities that are lined with the same ciliated mucous membranes as the nose. Sinuses empty into the nose through ostia (openings) located at the upper portion of the sinus cavity. Normally, sinus cilia are powerful enough to push mucus secretions upward against gravity and out of the osteal opening into the nose. When sinuses become infected, secretions are thickened and cilia become ineffective in draining secretions. Any condition that causes swelling in the nose and obstructs the ostia can cause sinusitis.

Allergy increases the risk of sinusitis, and allergic rhinitis is a common cause of sinusitis.

Primary symptoms of sinusitis include thick, purulent nasal discharge; postnasal drip; and cough. Patients may also experience headache, toothache, foul breath, and fever. Symptoms can be acute, lasting 7 to 10 days, or chronic, lasting for more than 3 months. Both acute and chronic sinusitis provoke asthma (National Heart, Lung, and Blood Institute [NHLBI]/World Health Organization [WHO], 2003).

All patients with asthma should be assessed for sinusitis because half of all people with asthma have evidence of sinusitis on x-ray. Treatment of sinusitis has been documented to improve asthma control (Tsao, Chen, Yeh, & Huang, 2003). Antibiotics are the appropriate treatment for sinusitis. Treatment needs to be prolonged to penetrate the bony paranasal sinus cavities and eradicate all bacteria. Primary care providers often underestimate the duration of antibiotic therapy. Typically a 10-day course of antibiotics is prescribed. Patients improve while on the 10-day course but symptoms return when the medication is completed. Short-course antibiotic therapy is insufficient to eradicate sinus infections and contributes to potential bacterial resistance. Antibiotic therapy for sinusitis needs to be for a 3-week duration.

Additional therapy is directed toward patient comfort. Intranasal saline washes can relieve nasal blockage and promote drainage of secretions, thus increasing comfort.

GASTROESOPHAGEAL REFLUX

GER is common in almost all age-groups. GER is passive transfer of gastric contents into the esophagus. Physiologic reflux occurs occasionally in everyone, typically after a large meal. Frequent, persistent reflux accompanied by complications distinguishes the occasional physiologic event from pathologic GER. Definitions of GER versus gastroe-sophageal reflux disease (GERD) vary depending on symptom severity or presence of tissue damage. Depending on the definition used, people with asthma may have GER or GERD. Reflux, whether GER or GERD has an impact on asthma and so the term "reflux" will be used to simplify the discussion.

The Asthma–Reflux Link

The tendency to develop respiratory symptoms after meals or when lying down was noted as early as the 12th century, but healthcare providers commonly overlook reflux as a cause or complication of asthma. Reflux can cause or aggravate asthma. People with reflux have impaired cough, swallow, and laryngeal closure reflexes. These impairments allow gastric contents to be aspirated into the respiratory tract. On the other hand, asthma and asthma treatment can cause reflux, so it is difficult to determine which condition causes the other in clinical practice. Although there is an ongoing debate about which condition causes which disease, it is critical to recognize symptoms of either disease and treat them appropriately. There are no studies to date that clearly establish the reflux-asthma association, but a wealth of clinical observation provides evidence that asthma control improves after medical or surgical treatment for reflux.

Incidence and Symptoms of Reflux

GER occurs in both children and adults with an overall incidence of about 8%. The incidence is much higher in people with asthma. Sixty percent to 80% of adults with asthma and 50% to 60% of children with asthma experience reflux (Wasowska-Królikowska, Toporowska-Kowalska, & Krogulska, 2002). In many of these people the reflux is silent. When reflux is not silent typical symptoms include heartburn, nausea, vomiting, acid taste in the pharynx, and dysphagia. Patients usually complain of discomfort after meals, after alcohol ingestion, when lying down, on exertion, and at night. Pulmonary symptoms include cough, wheeze, and dyspnea. Signs of reflux in infants include feeding resistance, fussiness, irritability, failure to thrive, apnea, choking, and recurrent vomiting.

Patients with asthma should be suspected of having reflux if they have any of the following: poor asthma control despite optimal therapy, no family history of asthma, no signs of allergy, new onset asthma as adults, or aggravation of pulmonary symptoms after use of bronchodilators. However, given how common reflux is in patients with asthma and the fact that it may be silent, the practitioner should keep a high index of suspicion for reflux in every person with asthma.

Theories of Reflux-Induced Bronchoconstriction

The esophagus and the bronchial tree have a common origin. Both developed from a common fetal tube and both have common vagal innervation. The normal function of the vagal nerve is thought to be that of a protective physiologic reflex to prevent airway exposure to acid. The current hypothesis with the most support is the vagal reflex theory. According to this theory, acid enters the esophagus and stimulates the vagal nerve terminals, which results in bronchoconstriction in the person with asthma. Microaspiration of gastric contents into the airway does lead to inflammatory changes, but this is thought to be less significant than the vagal theory (Wasowska-Królikowska et al., 2002).

Effect of Asthma on Reflux

The lower esophageal sphincter is a zone of low pressure rather than an actual sphincter. Infants commonly experience reflux because at birth the lower esophagus is positioned in the thoracic cavity and is subject to effects of negative intrathoracic pressures. As infants mature, the lower esophagus descends to the abdominal cavity, where higher intra-abdominal pressures around the esophageal sphincter prevent reflux. Asthma also creates conditions of negative pressure on the lower esophagus. Air trapping is common in asthma. This causes the diaphragm to descend and keeps the lower esopha-

gus exposed to negative pressure in the thoracic cavity. Coughing associated with asthma can increase intra-abdominal pressure, promoting reflux.

Asthma treatment can also cause reflux. Theophylline and systemically administered bronchodilators lower the pressure in the lower esophagus and stimulate acid production (NHLBI/WHO, 2003). Oral steroids have been reported to increase gastric acid contact times. The precise clinical significance of this effect is not known, but increased gastric acidity does correlate with respiratory symptoms (Lazenby, Guzzo, Harding, Patterson, Johnson, & Bradley, 2002). Fortunately, there is no evidence that inhaled bronchodilators cause reflux, so their use is not contraindicated in patients with asthma and reflux.

Diagnosis and Treatment of Reflux in the Person with Asthma

The diagnosis of reflux is based on a history of symptoms and is confirmed by 24-hour pH monitoring. There is currently no diagnostic test that can confirm reflux as the cause of asthma symptoms. Reflux as an asthma trigger should be suspected if respiratory symptoms are aggravated during a reflux episode.

Treatment is standard antireflux management. Behavioral management includes eating small, frequent meals and avoiding food or fluid intake 3 hours before bedtime. The head of the bed should be raised 6 to 8 inches. Foods that aggravate reflux, such as caffeinated beverages, alcohol, chocolate, and spicy and fatty foods, should be avoided. Patients who smoke should be counseled to stop smoking.

Pharmacotherapy includes the use of H2 blockers and proton pump inhibitors (PPIs). If H2 blockers are used they must be given in dosages that are two to four times the standard dosages. Currently, the PPIs are the most effective antireflux drugs. The PPIs omeprazole and lansoprazole have a shorter half-life in children than in adults, so higher weight-adjusted dosages are indicated in children (Gremse, 2004). The PPIs are safe and well tolerated.

Patients who fail to respond to medical treatment may be candidates for Nissen fundoplication surgery. This procedure entails surgically wrapping the upper stomach around the lower esophagus to create a zone of high pressure.

Generally, surgery is more effective in children than adults (Gremse, 2004). Although many clinical observations note improvement in asthma following treatment for reflux, scientific evidence is mixed. In a Cochrane review of scientific literature, antireflux treatment did not significantly improve lung function, symptoms, nocturnal asthma, or use of asthma medication, although subgroups did benefit (Gibson, Henry, & Coughlan, 2003). Others found that antireflux treatment did significantly improve pulmonary function and airway hyperresponsiveness (Jiang, Liang, Zeng, Liu, Liang, & Li, 2003) and decreased the use of asthma medication (Khoshoo, Le, Haydel, Landry, & Nelson, 2003).

THE NURSE'S ROLE IN EDUCATING THE PATIENT

Most people who present to the clinic for asthma care focus on symptoms related to difficulty breathing. Patients commonly lack understanding of the relationship between comorbid conditions associated with asthma and the control of asthma symptoms. The nurse can advocate for the patient by clearly explaining the relationship of the upper airway to the lower airway. Patients can appreciate basic explanations that the nose and throat are connected to the lower airway and that inflammation in the upper airway leads to inflammation in the lower airway. The nurse should clearly explain that symptom control of the upper airway leads to improved symptom control of asthma.

The most common condition associated with asthma is allergic rhinitis. Patients with both allergic rhinitis and asthma commonly question the need for multiple medications. As educator, the nurse has a vital role in explaining that allergy symptoms of itching, sneezing, and runny nose are caused by histamine release, whereas nasal congestion is caused by inflammation. When effects of antihistamines and anti-inflammatory medications are explained in relation to causative mechanisms, patient adherence to therapy increases. Another approach that is reassuring to patients is to explain that more medication is prescribed initially so that less medication is needed long term. As symptom control is achieved, medication dosages are reduced and possibly stopped altogether. Intranasal administration technique needs to be demonstrated and the patient should return the demonstration. Benefits of intranasal as opposed to oral administration need to be emphasized as well.

Sinusitis sufferers usually appreciate the need for antibiotic treatment, but commonly fail to understand the need for a 3-week course of therapy. The nurse educator's role is to explain the need to continue the complete course of antibiotics even after symptoms resolve.

The nurse as educator should review the relationship between GER and asthma with patients who have these conditions. Patients usually appreciate the need for antireflux medication, but need instruction regarding behavioral management of the disease.

SUMMARY

Allergic rhinitis, atopic dermatitis and asthma are recognized as the atopic triad because of many shared pathologies and symptom progression of these conditions in the same individuals. Atopic dermatitis shares many of the inflammatory features and triggers as asthma, and management principles parallel asthma management.

The relationship between asthma and allergic rhinitis has sufficient pathological links to warrant the label "united airway disease." Allergic rhinitis negatively impacts quality of life and healthcare costs and complicates the management of asthma. Pathophysiology, risk factors for the development of allergic rhinitis, theoretical links to asthma, triggers, clinical findings, classification, and management were discussed. Allergic rhinitis is a risk factor for sinusitis. The influence of sinus cavity anatomy to the development of sinusitis was reviewed as well as symptoms and principles of management and relation to asthma.

GER is common in people with asthma. Reflux is both caused by and causes asthma symptoms. Symptoms, treatment, approaches, and theories linking reflux to asthma were explored. The critical concept common to all associated conditions is that symptoms must be controlled for optimal asthma management. The nurse has a critical role in educating patients regarding the need to control symptoms relating to comorbid conditions.

CASE STUDY

A 14-year-old girl with moderate persistent asthma presents to the clinic complaining of exercise intolerance and waking in the middle of the night with cough since the weather turned cold. She denies other symptoms, but has signs of nasal congestion as evidenced by snuffing her nose and mouth breathing. She frequently rubs her nose despite denying itching. She responds that she has been taking the INSs that were prescribed on the last visit but complains that they "don't work." When asked if the intranasal spray runs out of her nose, she responds affirmatively. She reports that her congestion is worse in the morning and that drainage from her nose has been yellow-green for the past 3 weeks. She has been taking inhaled corticosteroids for asthma control but has not had the benefit from it that she enjoyed in the past. She has increased her use of albuterol in the last 3 weeks. On physical examination her nasal passages are pale and swollen, and they completely obstruct the airway.

Answer the following study questions, writing your responses on a separate sheet of paper. Compare your responses with the answers located at the end of the chapter.

1. What are the management goals for this patient?

2. How reliable is the history of no other symptoms beyond exercise intolerance and nocturnal cough?

3. What is the interpretation of the comment that the INSs "don't work?"

4. From what associated conditions does this girl suffer?

5. What are the priority teaching concepts for this visit?

Answers to Case Study

1. Management goals for this 14-year-old patient include reducing reliance on rescue medication and eliminating nocturnal and exercise-induced symptoms, itching, nasal drainage, and congestion.

2. The patient's subjective statement that she has no other symptoms is not reliable. Objective indicators of other symptoms are present, such as rubbing her nose, mouth breathing, and sniffling. Patients with chronic allergies tend to adapt to symptoms and become unaware of their presence.

3. INSs do work. However, they must penetrate the nasal mucosa to be effective. In the present case, the nasal cavities are completely obstructed and the medication runs out of the nose. The patient needs a short course of oral corticosteroids or a 3-day course of decongestant therapy to open the nasal passages so that the intranasal medication can be administered properly.

4. The patient suffers from allergic rhinitis as evidenced by nasal congestion and itching. The purulent nasal drainage indicates that she also

has sinusitis. She will need a 3-week course of antibiotics in addition to her other medications.

5. There are several priority teaching concepts. The patient needs to understand the relationship of allergic rhinitis and sinusitis to asthma control. She needs to appreciate the importance of limiting administration of decongestants to no more than 3 days. She also needs to understand that relief of swelling will allow proper administration of the INSs. Stress that the INSs are effective if administered properly. A return demonstration of proper administration of intranasal spray is essential. Finally, the patient needs to recognize increased use of albuterol as a sign that asthma is worsening and an indication that she should call her healthcare provider.

EXAM QUESTIONS

CHAPTER 12
Questions 69-79

69. Triggers that are more unique to atopic dermatitis than asthma are:

    a. pollens
    b. foods.
    c. viruses.
    d. mold.

70. United airway disease is a new concept that views upper and lower airway disease as

    a. one functioning airway with interrelated pathology.
    b. having separate unrelated pathological features.
    c. exclusively caused by allergic rhinitis.
    d. a precursor to progressive atopic dermatitis.

71. Allergic rhinitis from seasonal allergies is most commonly triggered by

    a. dust.
    b. pollen.
    c. exercise.
    d. strong odors.

72. According to research, early diagnosis and treatment of allergic conditions may

    a. have no impact on the course of the disease.
    b. eliminate the risk of asthma.
    c. increase the occurance of asthma.
    d. decrease the severity of asthma.

73. Typical symptoms in a person with allergic rhinitis include

    a. itchy, runny nose.
    b. purulent nasal drainage.
    c. fever.
    d. headache.

74. Principles of management of atopic dermatitis include

    a. developing a tolerance to unavoidable triggers.
    b. use of restraints to prevent scratching in young children.
    c. topical anti-inflammatory treatment.
    d. daily hygiene with antiseptic soaps.

75. The nurse should instruct the patient to administer intranasal medication by

    a. directing the spray away from the septum.
    b. directing the spray toward the septum.
    c. clearing the nose after administration.
    d. activating the spray as quickly as possible.

76. A complication of long-term use of intranasal decongestants is

    a. drowsiness.
    b. hypertension.
    c. nasal congestion.
    d. excessive nasal itching.

77. The only treatment that is capable of altering the course of allergic diseases is

    a. corticosteroid medication.

    b. anti-IgE therapy.

    c. combination therapy.

    d. immunotherapy.

78. The appropriate duration of antibiotic treatment for sinusitis is

    a. 7 days.

    b. 10 days.

    c. 14 days.

    d. 21 days.

79. The asthma treatment that is contraindicated in persons with GER is

    a. inhaled bronchodilator therapy.

    b. systemic bronchodilator therapy.

    c. inhaled corticosteroid therapy.

    d. anti-leukotriene therapy.

REFERENCES

Bosquet, J., van Cauwenberge, P,. & Khaltaev, N. (2001). Allergic rhinitis and its impact on asthma (ARIA) in collaboration with the World Health Organization (WHO). *Journal of Allergy and Clinical Immunology, 108*, (Suppl), S147-S336.

Boulay, M. & Boulet, L. (2003). The relationship between atopy, rhinitis and asthma: Pathophysiological considerations. *Current Opinion in Allergy and Clinical Immunology, 3*, 51-55.

Braunstahl, G. & Hellings, P. (2003). Allergic rhinitis and asthma: The link further unraveled. *Current Opinion in Pulmonary Medicine, 9*, 46-51.

Casale, T. & Dykewicz, M. (2004). Clinical implications of the allergic rhinitis–asthma link. *The American Journal of the Medical Sciences, 327*(3), 127-138.

Crystal-Peters, J., Neslusan, C., Crown, W,. & Torres, A. (2002). Treating allergic rhinitis in patients with comorbid asthma: The risk of asthma-related hospitalizations and emergency department visits, *Journal of Allergy and Clinical Immunology, 109*, 57-62.

Fuhlbrigge, A., & Adams, R. (2003). The effect of treatment of allergic rhinitis on asthma morbidity, including emergency department visits. *Current Opinion in Allergy and Clinical Immunology, 3*, 29-32.

Gibson, P., Henry, R., & Coughlan, J. (2003). *Gastro-esophageal reflux treatment for asthma in adults and children.* Retrieved December 19, 2004, from Cochrane Database of Systematic Reviews

Gremse, D. (2004). GERD in the pediatric patient: Management considerations. *Medscape General Medicine, 6*(2). Retrieved May 12, 2004, from http://www.medscape.com/viewarticle/472765

Helm, R. (2004). Diet and the development of atopic disease. *Current Opinion in Allergy and Clinical Immunology, 4*, 125-129.

Jiang, S, Liang, R., Zeng, Z., Liu, Q, Liang, Y., & Li, J. (2003). Effects of antireflux treatment on bronchial hyperresponsiveness and lung function in asthmatic patients with GERD. *World Journal of Gastroenterology, 9*(5), 1233-1235.

Khoshoo, V., Le, T., Haydel, R., Landry, L., & Nelson, C. (2003). Role of gastroesophageal reflux in older children with persistent asthma. *Chest, 123*(4), 1008-1013.

Koh, Y. & Kim, C. (2003). The development of asthma in patients with allergic rhinitis. *Current Opinion in Allergy and Clinical Immunology, 3*, 159-164.

Lazenby, J., Guzzo, M., Harding, S., Patterson, P., Johnson, L., & Bradley, L. (2002). Oral corticosteroids increase esophageal acid contact times in patients with stable asthma. *Chest, 121*(2), 625-634.

Leung, D., Boguniewicz, M., Howell, M., Nomura, I., & Hamid, Q. (2004). New insights into atopic dermatitis. *Journal of Clinical Investigation, 113*, 651-657.

Murray, J. & Rusznak, C. (2003). Asthma and rhinosinusitis. *Current Opinion in Otolaryngology & Head and Neck Surgery, 11*, 49-53.

National Heart, Lung, and Blood Institute/World Health Organization. (2003). *Global initiative for asthma: Global strategy for asthma management and prevention.* (NIH Publication No. 02-3659). Retrieved September 12, 2002, from http://www.ginasthma.com

Pascual, J. & Fleischer, A. (2004). Tacrolimus ointment (Protopic) for atopic dermatitis. *Skin Therapy Letter, 9*(9), 1-5. Retrieved December 15, 2004, from http://www.medscape.com/viewarticle/495046_print

Pawankar, R. (2004). Allergic rhinitis and asthma: the link, the new ARIA classification and global approaches to treatment. *Current Opinion in Allergy and Clinical Immunology, 4*, 1-4.

Taramarcaz, P. & Gibson, P. (2003). *Intranasal corticosteroids for asthma control in people with coexisting asthma and rhinitis.* Retrieved November 29, 2004, from Cochrane Database of Systematic Reviews.

Tsao, C., Chen, L., Yeh, K., & Huang, J. (2003). Concomitant chronic sinusitis treatment in children with mild asthma: The effect on bronchial hyperresponsiveness. *Chest, 123*(3), 757-764.

U.S. Food and Drug Administration. (2005). *FDA public health advisory: Elidel (pimecrolimus) cream and protopic (tacrolimus) ointment.* Retrieved March 19, 2005, from www.fda.gov.cder/drug/advisory/elidel_protopic.htm

Wasowska-Królikowska, K., Toporowska-Kowalska, E., & Krogulska, A. (2002). Asthma and gastroesophageal reflux in children. *Medical Science Monitor, 8*(3), RA64-71.

CHAPTER 13

THE NURSE AS ASTHMA EDUCATOR

CHAPTER OBJECTIVE

Upon completion of this chapter, the reader will recognize asthma education as a critical component of comprehensive asthma management and identify appropriate asthma teaching content and strategies in various clinical contexts.

LEARNING OBJECTIVES

After studying this chapter, the reader will be able to

1. identify five national goals for patient education about asthma and recognize current gaps in reaching those goals.

2. identify five components of a comprehensive asthma education plan.

3. identify appropriate asthma education content for sequential healthcare visits.

4. recognize urgent care visits as teachable moments.

5. identify four appropriate methods of teaching asthma content.

6. recognize five potential health outcomes of asthma education.

7. identify three components of culturally competent asthma education.

8. recognize methods of evaluating the effectiveness of clinical teaching.

9. recognize two benefits of asthma educator certification.

OVERVIEW

Previous chapters reviewed the epidemiology, pathophysiology, diagnosis, monitoring, and management of asthma as well as unique lifespan issues and comorbid conditions associated with asthma. These concepts provide the nurse with a foundation for providing patients and families with quality asthma education. This chapter focuses on the content and process of patient- and family-centered asthma education.

Asthma is a very controllable disease, but control requires patient and family involvement. By nature, asthma is a variable disease. Symptoms are constantly changing in response to the weather, exposure to environmental triggers, and changes in the individual such as growth. This variability demands frequent adjustments in the patient's treatment plan. Recognition of early warning signs and prompt treatment are key to asthma control. Optimal control can only be achieved if the patient and family are educated to make sound management decisions. Suboptimal control results in excessive and costly healthcare utilization and poor quality of life for asthma sufferers.

Because education is critical to optimal asthma outcomes, experts have mandated that healthcare providers include education in every treatment plan.

The National Asthma Education and Prevention Program (NAEPP, 1997) placed higher priority on asthma education by including education at every patient interaction. Despite efforts to promote asthma education, many primary care providers fail to incorporate the guidelines into practice.

Nurses are in ideal positions to fill the gap in patient education. Nurses generally have the advantage of having time to spend with the patient, and patients report that they are comfortable talking to nurses. The nurse has a unique opportunity to profoundly change the lives of people with asthma by providing asthma education that is supportive and tailored to individual patient and family needs.

GOALS OF ASTHMA EDUCATION

The National Heart, Lung, and Blood Institute (NHLBI) in association with the World Health Organization (WHO) (2003) have identified goals of asthma education. Asthma education aims to provide the patient and family with appropriate information and training so that the patient can keep well and make sound treatment decisions. An ongoing patient-family partnership with the health team is an essential component of education. Education should increase understanding, skills, satisfaction, and confidence so that adherence and self-management is increased.

Unfortunately, asthma management goals are falling far short of the NAEPP's goals. Recently, the largest and most comprehensive survey about children and asthma to date, Children and Asthma in America, revealed disturbing findings (Asthma in America, 2004). In-depth telephone interviews were conducted with 800 families of children with asthma. More than half of all children with asthma had a severe attack in the past year and 27% had an attack so severe they thought their life was in danger. The findings from the survey as compared to the NAEPP's goals are listed in Table 13-1.

Data from this survey indicate that many children with asthma are in poor control. The majority of parents in the survey disagreed with the child's perception of symptoms. The disturbing findings in this study were attributed, in part, to ineffective parent-child communication. The study recommended that parents regularly ask their child about symptoms.

Especially disturbing is the fact that respondents reported never hearing of the two major causes of underlying asthma symptoms: tightening of airway smooth muscles (90%) or inflammation (93%). Only 53% of children with severe asthma and 63% of those with moderate asthma reported using daily controller medication in the past 4 weeks. Thirty percent incorrectly identified quick-relief medication as long-term controller medication.

The Asthma in America (1998) survey also interviewed adults with asthma and 700 physicians. Findings among adults were similar to the child study results, indicating that asthma is out of control for many patients. Although physicians reported that they are following national guidelines, levels of care do not meet current standards. Furthermore, 71% of the adults with asthma who participated in the survey stated that there was a need for more patient education about asthma.

COMPONENTS OF COMPREHENSIVE ASTHMA EDUCATION

The components of asthma education are defined by the NAEPP (1997) and have been expanded upon by the international Global Initiative for Asthma (GINA) (NHLBI/WHO, 2003).

The NAEPP guidelines clearly establish that asthma education begins at the time of diagnosis and is reinforced at every opportunity. The involvement of the primary care provider in patient education sends a clear message that education is important. However, education involves all mem-

TABLE 13-1: FINDINGS FROM THE CHILDREN AND ASTHMA IN AMERICA SURVEY COMPARED TO THE NAEPP GOALS

NAEPP's Goals	Children and Asthma in America Survey
Minimal or no symptoms	In the past 4 weeks: 67% of children reported day, night, and exercise-induced symptoms; 19% reported having symptoms three times per week to daily; 22% reported nocturnal symptoms once per week
Minimal or no exacerbations, including hospitalizations and emergency room (ER) visits	23% had visits to the ER in the past year; 42% reported unscheduled acute care visits in past year
No activity limitations; no missed school or work	54% missed school in past year, with an average of 4 days/child; 39% of parents missed work due to child's asthma; 62% reported activity limitation
Minimal use of short-acting beta-agonist (rescue inhaler)	42% of children who used rescue medication in the past 4 weeks, used it three times per week to once daily; 26% used it daily
Have a written action plan	54% of all children said they did not have a written asthma action plan
Visit healthcare provider two times per year	25% reported no visit in the last year; 54% did not have a lung function test in the past year

Note. From Asthma in America. (2004). Children and Asthma in America. Retrieved December 21, 2004, from http://www.asthmainamerica.com/children_index.html

bers of the team and, as mentioned above, the nurse commonly has time to spend with patients and is perceived as approachable.

KEY EDUCATION CONCEPTS

Basic Facts About Asthma

Key asthma education concepts are listed in Table 13-2. The concept, "basic facts about asthma" refers to providing the patient and family with an understanding of the underlying pathophysiology of asthma. This is best accomplished in simple terms with visual aides. The three main features of an asthma attack are described as airway swelling, narrowing (or tightening), and mucus accumulation.

Colored illustrations can enhance the discussion, but in the author's experience a nonthreatening three-dimensional model, such as Radical Randy,™ is most effective (Meng & McConnell, 2003). Radical Randy™ is a lifelike model whose right chest opens to show healthy airways. Miniature three-dimensional airways allow for demonstration of optimal airflow. When the child grasps the basic concepts of airway anatomy and airflow, the left chest is opened. The left chest reveals angry, red, inflamed airways that are choked by tight smooth muscles. A second miniature airway is inflated to demonstrate swelling and tightening of smooth muscles around the inflamed airway and loss of airway diameter, which results in diminished airflow. The most appealing feature to children is the artificial green mucus that is added to the inflamed airway. Symptoms of an acute attack can easily be described with the model. Children understand how coughing, wheezing, and tight chest are related to the model of the inflamed lung. An anxious facial

TABLE 13-2: KEY ASTHMA EDUCATION CONCEPTS FOR PATIENTS AND FAMILIES

Basic Facts about Asthma

- The contrast between inflamed and healthy airways
- What happens to the airways during an asthma attack

Roles of Medication

- How medications work
  - Long-term controllers: prevent symptoms by reducing inflammation
  - Rescue medications: quick acting; relax airway smooth muscles
- Emphasize the importance of long-term controller medication and not to expect immediate relief

Skills

- Inhaler (metered-dose inhaler or dry powdered inhalers) use with return demonstration
- Spacer and holding chamber use
- Symptom monitoring: recognition of early warning signs, peak flow meter use

Environmental Control Measures

- Identifying and avoiding triggers

When and how to take rescue actions

- Responding to changes in asthma severity

Note. From National Asthma Education and Prevention Program. (1997). Expert panel report 2. *Guidelines for the diagnosis and management of asthma.* (NIH Publication No. 97-4051). Bethesda, MD: National Institutes of Health, National Heart, Lung, and Blood Institute. Available online at www.nhlbi.nih.gov/guidelines/asthma/index.pdf

overlay links children's feelings of anxiety to pathological events in the airway.

This model has facilitated children's understanding of abstract concepts such as inflammation and bronchoconstriction in a manner that words or pictures cannot express. Radical Randy™ was designed for teaching children ages 7 through 12, but parents who have seen the model in clinic sometimes ask for the clinician to use the model to facilitate their own understanding. Field tests demonstrated that the model was effective in increasing children's knowledge and that children preferred learning with Radical Randy.™ The model is available through Legacy Products, Inc. (www.legacyproductsinc.com)

Roles of Medication

Patients and families need to understand how to use the two classes of asthma medication: the long-term controllers and the quick-relief medications. This is perhaps the most challenging concept to teach because proper use of asthma medications is inconsistent with the patient and family's logic and past history of medication use. Typically, patients expect to use medication when they are ill. They expect prompt relief and discontinuation of the medication when symptoms abate.

Proper use of asthma medication does not fit this logic. Patients and families need to understand that prevention is key and controllers (inhaled corticosteroids) need to be taken every day, even when the patient is not experiencing symptoms. The patient and family need to be adivsed to expect a delayed response that may take several weeks. Patients should be assured that if taken every day, controller medication is effective. Quick-relief medication gives prompt relief of symptoms. Patients commonly perceive that quick-relief medication "works." This belief reinforces overuse of quick-relief medication. This is a dangerous practice for two reasons. Controller medication is abandoned and inflammation goes unchecked. Furthermore, repeated use of quick-relief medication down regulates the beta-agonist receptor sites. Quick relief medication eventually becomes ineffective. Patients sometimes understand loss of effect as developing "tolerance" to the medication.

Despite teaching, it is estimated that only 50% of patients use controller medication as prescribed (NHLBI/WHO, 2003). This represents an education failure and supports the recommendation to review and reinforce medication administration concepts at every visit. Adherence increases if patients and families accept the diagnosis, recognize that asthma is serious, and feel in control.

Skills

Asthma skills include use of asthma devices: nebulizers, metered-dose inhalers (MDIs), dry powdered inhalers (DPIs), spacers, and peak flow meters.

Nebulizers are simple to operate. A one-time explanation is usually sufficient for accurate operation of the device. Families should be given a written set of operating instructions and directions for cleaning the nebulizer. MDIs, DPIs, and peak flow meters require different inhalation maneuvers. Patients who use all three devices tend to become confused. The nurse should carefully assess the patient's ability to accurately perform the required maneuvers. Difficulty managing different techniques calls for simplification of the treatment plan. For example, use of the peak flow meter may have to be sacrificed if the patient is confused about inhalation techniques between the peak flow meter and the MDI.

Peak flow technique is described in chapter 4; MDI and spacer technique are described in chapter 5. Each DPI operates differently, depending on the manufacturer. The reader is referred to manufacturer's literature for the use of DPIs.

Accurate MDI and spacer, or DPI technique is critical to asthma control. Poor technique results in limited medication delivery to the lungs and ineffective asthma control. Failure to use a spacer is a common error. Cost or hassle of carrying a bulky device may also be issues for the patient. Adherence is increased for children if they keep a second spacer at school. Explain to patients that they will use more medication with less effect without a spacer and that this is ultimately more expensive than not using a spacer.

Every patient, regardless of ability to demonstrate accurate inhaler technique, has a tendency to deteriorate in skill proficiency over time. Patients should be instructed to bring medications to each clinic visit and demonstrate inhaler technique at every visit. Correct or reinforce technique as needed.

Environmental Control Measures

Individual's unique triggers need to be identified, but this is difficult for most patients, especially for those sensitized to perennial triggers such as dust. Signs of allergy to house dust mites are nasal congestion and stuffiness early in the morning. This sign is a marker for the need for education on dust control measures. However, most persons with asthma are allergic to dust, so it is appropriate to assume that all patients would benefit from dust control measures. Highest concentrations of dust mites are found in bedding. Educational focus should be on eliminating dust from the bedroom. (See chapter 6 for dust control measures.)

Environmental tobacco smoke is avoidable, but motivation to stop smoking may be lacking. Upon questioning, smoking is commonly denied but is evident from findings on home visits and results of studies that measure urinary cotinine (a marker for nicotine in the urine). A suggested strategy is to phrase the assessment question, "Who smokes in the house?" rather than "Does anyone smoke in the house?" Include assessment of smoking in secondary residences of children from broken families. The goal of education is smoking cessation. Families need to understand how damaging active and passive smoking is to the lungs. (See chapter 6 for smoking control measures.) Children report that it is difficult to ask adults to stop smoking. Occasionally, children's requests to the adults in their lives have been met with physical violence. It is recommended that the healthcare provider, rather than the child, deliver the stop smoking message.

Patients should be asked what symptoms they experience after exposure to other triggers, such as weather change, animals, pollen, mold, strong odors, or emotional upset. Patients may initially have difficulty responding to these questions. The asthma educator should explain that asking these questions heightens awareness of responses to triggers and encourages future identification. Trigger avoidance strategies should be tailored to the patient's specific triggers. Some patients may benefit from allergy testing. Education is directed to triggers that are positively identified on the allergy test.

Note that exercise is not included in the trigger list. Exercise is best conceptualized as an early warning sign of worsening asthma. Classification as a trigger sends an erroneous message that exercise is to be avoided. Patients should be instructed to report increasing activity intolerance to the healthcare provider.

Responding to Changes in Asthma Severity

Asthma is like the weather—it is always changing. The use of the weather metaphor helps patients and families conceptualize the variable nature of asthma. Like altering activity plans or amount of clothing for changes in the weather, asthma medication is altered according to changes in asthma severity.

Adjusting medication requires sophisticated decision-making. Patients and families need time to become familiar with a basic understanding of asthma before assuming responsibility of self-management with medication dosing adjustments. Telephone numbers with 24-hour access to healthcare providers are given to families so the provider can initially guide the patient and family in medica-

tion adjustment decisions. Over the course of the next several clinic visits, the patient and family are assessed for decision-making ability. Individual ability is reflected in level of decisions that are incorporated to the personal self-management plan.

All patients need to recognize early warning signs of worsening asthma. They should administer quick-relief medication on an as-needed basis only. They should recognize that increasing the frequency of use of quick-relief medication warrants a clinic visit to reevaluate asthma severity. Depending upon decision-making ability, patients and families are taught to increase controller medication when asthma symptoms increase. Also, depending upon ability, patients and families can be taught to gradually decrease controller medication in a stepwise fashion when no asthma symptoms are experienced for at least a 2-month period. If control is maintained, the step down process can be carefully continued. The patient and family are instructed to quickly increase controller medication at the first sign of worsening symptoms. The adage, "fast up, slow down" may help the patient remember. Specific dosage changes are determined by the primary care provider and written on the individualized action plan (see chapter 14). The asthma educator should incorporate the action plan into the teaching session.

Based on the findings of the Asthma Action America® survey, parents should be taught to communicate with children about symptoms and vice versa. Lack in parent-child communication may stem from the fact that children spend a majority of the day in school, away from working parents. Children, by nature, attempt to normalize their lives, which commonly means ignoring asthma symptoms. The educator should give children the clear message to tell an adult when they have symptoms. Parents cannot assume that the child will report symptoms, but should spend a moment reviewing how the child's breathing was over the course of the day.

A STEPWISE APPROACH TO PATIENT EDUCATION

Asthma is a complex topic. Providing all education at one visit can easily overwhelm the patient and family. Both the NAEPP (1997) and GINA (2003) guidelines delineate approaches for providing asthma education in a stepwise approach. The GINA recommendations stress essential components that are presented in Table 13-3. According to the GINA guidelines, the patient needs information about the diagnosis, simple information about available treatments, and explanations of the recommended treatments at the initial visit. For example, the parent of a 1-year-old child who is relying on nebulizer treatments should be shown an MDI with spacer and facemask. The nurse should demonstrate how the MDI and spacer are used and explain that drug delivery is more accurate, easier, and efficient with the device. Ideally, the parent will participate in the choice to change methods. Participation may take the form of gradually weaning the child from the nebulizer to the MDI and spacer.

Patients should be given the opportunity to express their expectations about asthma and its treatment. Usually the healthcare provider needs to raise expectations about benefits of therapy because patients assume that some symptoms are acceptable. The patient should receive a clear message that goals of therapy include no nocturnal symptoms, no missed work or school, no emergency room (ER) visits, full participation in activities (including sports), the best possible lung function, and minimal side effects from medication.

Patients should have an opportunity to express fears and concerns. A common concern is steroid phobia. It is important to address this issue, even if the concern is not expressed by the patient because corticosteroids are the mainstay of asthma treatment. The educator should differentiate anabolic steroids that are sometimes abused by athletes from corticosteroids used for therapy. The safety and

TABLE 13-3: INDIVIDUALIZING EDUCATION IN A STEPWISE MANNER

Goal: To provide the patient and family with suitable training so that the patient can remain well and adjust treatment according to a medication plan developed with the healthcare provider.

Key Components

- Development of a partnership
- Acceptance of asthma as a chronic disease
- Information sharing
- Full discussion of expectations
- Expression of fears and concerns

The patient then requires information about:

- Diagnosis
- Difference between "rescue" and "controller" medication
- Prevention measures
- Early warning signs of worsening asthma and actions to take
- Training in monitoring asthma
- How and when to seek medical attention

The patient then requires:

- A guided self-management plan
- Regular supervision, revision, reward, and reinforcement

Note. From National Heart, Lung and Blood Institute/World Health Organization. (2003). *Global initiative for asthma: Global strategy for asthma management and prevention.* (NIH Publication No. 02-3659). Retrieved December 24, 2004, from http://www.ginasthma.com

advantage of inhaled delivery with deposition of small dosages directly to the lungs should be stressed.

The NAEPP recommendations for stepwise education are more comprehensive than the GINA recommendations. The NAEPP recommendations are listed in Table 13-4. Sample assessment questions, teaching content, and skills for the initial and each subsequent visit are delineated. In addition to content, the NAEPP recommendations stress assessment. Effective teaching is always based on assessment. Assessment enables the educator to adjust the information to the individual, needs, concerns and education level. Content adjusted to these needs is meaningful to the patient and is retained longer. Assessment is also conducted in a stepwise approach, with initial focus on worries, concerns, and expectations and later focus on issues or concerns implementing the treatment plan.

Not all patients need all education components. For example, patients with mild asthma do not need to use peak flow meters, and patients with stable asthma will usually not adhere to peak flow instructions. It is important to tailor the education, provide it in steps, and periodically review understanding.

Verbal information should be supplemented with written information (or pictorial for low literacy patients). Patients should be told to take note of any questions and to bring them to the next visit. All teaching should be documented in the medical record.

Teachable Moments

Patients may be more receptive to asthma education after a severe asthma exacerbation. Hospitalization in the past 12 months, especially intensive care admission with intubation, is an indicator of fatality prone asthma. It is estimated that 74% of hospital admissions are preventable (NHLBI/WHO, 2003).

Any person with asthma who presents to the ER or is hospitalized is a priority candidate for education. Priority topics include identifying and avoiding the trigger that caused the acute exacerbation, correct use of medications, and importance of close medical supervision in the immediate period following the exacerbation. (See chapter 10 for more information.)

METHODS OF TEACHING

In addition to individual teaching, asthma education is delivered by written material, video programs, group sessions, camp programs, or computer packages. None of these methods

replaces individual sessions with the primary health care providers (NAEPP, 1997); rather, they are a supplement to provider education. Selection of a teaching method should be based on established program outcomes rather than patient preference because patient preference does not always translate into effective learning (NHLBI/WHO, 2003).

It has not always been possible to determine which component of education is the most effective because most patients receive a combination of approaches. What is probably effective is to give information verbally and then reinforce it with several other methods. Programs that give information only increase knowledge but do not always improve outcomes. The combination of personalized advice with interactive learning opportunities, such as sessions conducted by specially trained nurses, group classes, and support groups, does impact outcomes. Adolescents have unique adherence issues that may be best met through support groups. Videotapes have been shown to be particularly effective in teaching good inhaler technique.

Only qualified asthma educators should teach formal programs (NAEPP, 1997). Developed programs should not be modified in the interest of saving time. They should be delivered as designed to maintain validity.

Children

Programs for children are designed for the school-age child. These take the form of school-based programs or camp programs (see chapter 15 for a description of a camp program). These programs focus on prevention and management of attacks and are usually interactive in nature. An example is Open Airways, a school-based asthma education program targeting minority children ages 8 to 11. It is available through the American Lung Association and has been translated into Spanish. The Starbright® Foundation has an interactive CD-ROM, *Quest for the Code*, designed for children ages 7 to 15 and is available in English and Spanish.

TABLE 13-4: RECOMMENDED ASTHMA TEACHING CONTENT BY VISIT

Assessment Questions	Teaching Content	Skills
Initial Visit Focus on the patient's: • Concerns • Quality of life • Expectations • Goals of treatment	Teach in simple language	Teach and demonstrate
"What worries you most about your asthma?" "What do you want to accomplish at this visit?" "What do you want to be able to do that you can't do now?" "What do you expect from treatment?" "What medicines have you tried?" "What other questions do you have for me today?"	What is asthma? Asthma as a chronic disease Explanation of how airways become swollen (inflammation), narrow, and filled with mucus Asthma treatments: Long-term controller and quick-acting rescue medications When to seek medical advice Provide contact telephone number	Inhaler and spacer technique and return demonstration Link self-monitoring skills to an action plan Recognize intensity and frequency of symptoms Review signs of worsening asthma: – nocturnal cough –exercise intolerance –increased use of rescue medication
Recommendations for first follow-up visit Focus (same as above) "What medications are you taking?" "How and when are you taking them?" "What problems have you had taking your medications?" "Please show me how you use your inhaled medication."	Use of two types of medications Evaluation of progress in asthma control using symptoms and peak flow as a guide	Revisions and use of self-management plan Revision and use of action plan Peak flow monitoring and recording Correct inhaler and spacer or dry powdered inhaler (DPI) technique
Recommendations for second follow up visit Focus on: quality of life, goals of treatment, medications, and expectations of visit "Have you noticed anything in your home, school or work that makes your asthma worse?" "Describe for me how you know to call your doctor or go to the hospital for asthma care." "What questions do you have about the action plan?" "Can we make it easier?" "Are your medications causing you any problems?"	How to identify exposures that cause or make asthma worse How to control house dust mites and animal exposures, if applicable Avoidance of active and passive smoke Review of all medications Review and interpretation of PEFR or symptom diaries.	Inhaler and spacer or DPI technique Revisions and use of self-management plan Review of PEFR technique Revision and use of action plan Confirmation that the patient knows what to do if asthma gets worse
Recommendations for all subsequent follow up visits Focus: same as 2nd visit "How have you tried to control things that make your asthma worse?" "Please show me how you use your inhaled medication."	Review and reinforcement of all educational messages	Same as second visit

Note. From National Asthma Education and Prevention Program. (1997). Expert panel report 2. *Guidelines for the diagnosis and management of asthma.* (NIH Publication No. 97-4051). Bethesda, MD: National Institutes of Health, National Heart, Lung, and Blood Institute. Available online at www.nhlbi.nih.gov/guidelines/asthma/index.pdf

Adolescents

Adolescents are interested in learning ways of coping with asthma and knowing the experiences of other teens. Adverse events, such as death of a peer from asthma or hospitalization with intubation, are disturbing to teens. Networking with peers should be directed toward others who are coping well.

Emotional support is a major issue. Adolescents expect support from the healthcare provider. Adolescents have many demands of the educator. They expect the educator to be sensitive, create a positive atmosphere, possess good communication skills, and understand adolescent development. They want to be listened to and have their opinions heard. They are motivated for educational sessions when they receive the agenda in advance. Advanced information allows them to become familiar with the content and timing of the program and allows them time to prepare. Adolescents want an active role in education and problem solving information in terms that they can understand. Adolescents are part of the computer generation. They are puzzled when computers are not used for education (Kyngäs, 2003).

Adults

Education for adults is usually conducted on an individual basis. Experts believe this method is the most effective strategy for adult education (Janson et al., 2003). Studies have shown that adults benefit more from clinic visits when they are taught how to give information to the healthcare provider in a clear manner. They also benefit when they are taught information seeking techniques and methods of checking their understanding of what the provider told them. These strategies also increase adherence (NHLBI/WHO, 2003).

CULTURALLY COMPETENT ASTHMA EDUCATION

Minority groups in the United States are over-represented low-income populations—populations with higher prevalence of disease and more barriers to accessing healthcare. Illiteracy and poor English skills are high among these groups and complicate healthcare delivery. However, when culturally competent care and education is provided, health outcomes among minority groups improve. The challenge to the nurse is to understand culturally competent education and integrate cultural concepts into practice.

Culturally Oriented Beliefs

Patients' beliefs about asthma and asthma treatment must be considered for successful education outcomes. Cultural groups vary in their health beliefs, and these variations commonly conflict with traditional medical beliefs. Failure to recognize these differences leads to distrust and creates distance between the patient and the provider. The practice of many healthcare providers is consistent with the Health Belief Model (Rosenstock, Strecher, & Becker, 1988). That is, a person's health behavior is based on his or her perception of their vulnerability for illness and their perception of the advantages and disadvantages of treatment. This model is based on decision-making as a culturally important concept. The Health Belief Model is consistent with the focus of the NAEPP's education goals. This model is useful in mainstream American culture; however, the model is not useful in cultures where community decision-making is valued, such as in many Asian cultures (George, 2001). In these instances, it may be more effective to consider partnership with the community.

Cultural beliefs may affect the way the patient interacts with the healthcare provider. A primary goal of asthma management is to develop partnerships with patients and families. For some patients, however, cultural beliefs may deter the patient from interacting with the healthcare provider as a peer. Asking questions may be viewed as challenging the provider. Lack of asking questions should not be interpreted as lack of interest. The flexible educator should anticipate questions and actively determine if the anticipated questions are a concern for the patient.

Culture also influences decision-making power within the family and thus has implications for identification of whom to include in patient education. Traditional western culture identifies the patient and their caregiver as the focus of education, but this may not be appropriate for all patients. In some cultures, the husband or father is the decision-maker whereas the wife or mother is the caretaker. Among the Southeast Asian Hmong people, traditionally the family or clan elder is the decision-maker. Extended families are important in Hispanic communities (George, 2001). The nurse can make sound decisions for inclusion of appropriate family members by identifying how the family is defined, whether group or individual decisions are valued, and who makes decisions.

Cultural beliefs affect perception of treatment. Harmless beliefs that have meaning to the family should be incorporated into care, but harmful practices need to be modified in a sensitive fashion. A common belief related to asthma treatment among Hispanic groups is that presence of a chihuahua in the home will cure the child of asthma. In reality, the chihuahua has a predisposition to develop respiratory illness as it ages. Children, on the other hand, tend to experience a lessening of asthma symptoms as they age. There is no association between owning a chihuahua and childhood asthma, but the belief is harmless and can safely be incorporated into the care plan. A common Mexican asthma remedy is the use of oregano tea. The active ingredient in the tea is similar to the methylxanthine class of drugs. Theophylline is a methylxanthine and has bronchodilator effects. Although the oregano tea proba-

bly has some beneficial effects, other medications are more effective. Sole reliance on tea may be dangerous. Using the tea may be valued as a family or cultural tradition, or it may be the family's only option because of limited finances. The nurse educator should explore the meaning of the remedy with the family and determine resources available to help the family obtain appropriate medication.

Cultural beliefs may differ among rural versus urban populations. A common asthma related tradition among southern rural people is to make a hatch mark on a tree. When the child with asthma grows to the hatch mark, he will no longer have asthma. This belief is probably rooted in the misperception that children "outgrow" their asthma, but it is conceptualized in terms that have meaning to rural patients. The nurse educator should address the patient's logic to increase understanding. In this case, the hatch mark can be incorporated into teaching by using it to represent a symbol of reaching adult height. Affirm that many children do have a lessening of symptoms as they reach the hatch mark but explain that asthma never completely goes away.

Folk tales and story telling may be appropriate methods of instruction for Hispanic or African American minority groups with strong oral traditions (George, 2001). See chapter 14 for use of fairy tales and story telling in a skit format with children.

Language

Whenever possible, the nurse should ensure that asthma education is conducted in the patient and family's native language by someone fluent in the language. Using family members as translators may result in inaccurate translation or block communication by disrupting the power structure in the family. However, the nurse who is not fluent in the patient's language can build rapport by making the effort to communicate in the patient's language by using familiar phrases.

Verbal instruction should be reinforced with written material in the patient's native language. This is a challenge because the predominant immigrant groups, Southeast Asians and Hispanics, speak many different dialects and subgroups are sensitive to differences in dialect. Some institutions are recruiting certified translators who are fluent in the predominant dialect of the area served by the institution. A second certified translator should review translated educational materials to confirm their accuracy.

Literacy

Approximately 25% of the adult population of the United States is functionally illiterate (Doak & Doak, 1996). Inability to read causes embarrassment, so the nurse should avoid direct questions about reading ability. Inability to read can be assessed by noting the patient's preference for pictorial over printed material, lack of note taking, or use of excuses such as, "I left my glasses at home." Written material should be at the fifth or sixth grade level and include many pictures. Programs should use alternative modes to reading, such as videotapes, discussion, and interactive skills training.

POTENTIAL BENEFITS OF ASTHMA EDUCATION

Successful asthma programs are based on sound understanding of the theory of behavior change. They also incorporate strategies proven to increase knowledge, skills, and confidence. Such programs have reduced morbidity and excessive healthcare utilization among adults with asthma (Wolf, Guevara, Grum, Clark, & Cates, 2002). Education for adults without action plans, self-monitoring, or regular follow-up visits has no impact on asthma outcomes. Symptom monitoring is as effective as peak flow monitoring, and regular follow-up leads to reduced morbidity and improved lung function (Powell & Gibson, 2002). Other benefits of adult self-management programs include significantly

reduced hospitalizations and ER visits, fewer missed work days, fewer nocturnal symptoms, and improved quality of life. These effects were most apparent when programs included written self-management plans (Gibson et al., 2002).

Individual face-to-face teaching appears to be the most effective teaching strategy with adults. A study showed that 30-minute individual teaching sessions with advanced nurse practitioners that focused on basic pathology and the use of medication and used models and illustrations resulted in improved asthma control. The teaching was designed to simulate an actual clinic encounter. Patients were given written action plans based on their individual peak flow zones. Adherence with controller therapy increased 30% and adults' perceived control of asthma increased (Janson et al., 2003).

Programs that include strategies for preventing and managing asthma attacks in children have improved physiologic functioning and confidence and decreased the number of missed school days, ER visits, and activity limitations. Programs are effective with children of all severity levels but tend to be especially effective among children with more severe asthma. Programs with adequate follow up generally show greater effectiveness than programs with inadequate follow-up (Wolf, Guevara, Grum, Clark, & Cates, 2002).

Many of the child asthma programs are targeted toward low-income minority groups because these groups are less likely to receive primary care and because acute healthcare utilization is especially high. When interactive seminars were targeted to primary care providers, low-income families benefited. Families' use of controller medication and action plans increased and children missed less school. Effective teaching and communication gave families more confidence and less worry. Clarity of communication provided a picture of how the treatment plan could help the child reach management goals. These findings point to the need for improved teaching and communication strategies between healthcare providers and low-income families (Brown, Bratton, Cabana, Kaciroti, & Clark, 2004).

Combined approaches are also effective. A program used in low-income Detroit elementary schools used a combination of Open Airways (a four week asthma education program designed by the American Lung Association for school children to teach self-management), environmental control classes, environmental building assessment with remediation suggestions, and strategies for increasing communication with physicians which resulted in positive outcomes. Children were more aware of symptoms and reported symptoms more frequently. Parents took more steps to manage asthma. Science grades improved and school absences decreased. Results were evident for 2 years after the intervention (Clark et al., 2004).

EVALUATION METHODS FOR CLINICAL TEACHING

Each follow-up clinic visit provides the asthma educator with the opportunity to evaluate the effectiveness of patient and family education. Most of the evaluation data are obtained by subjective reports from the patient and family. Each patient should be assessed for urgent acute care visits, ER visits, hospitalizations, activity tolerance, and missed work or school days since the last visit. Improvements in these outcomes are linked to effective education.

Physical findings are commonly misleading, but improvement in pulmonary function is a reliable objective indicator of asthma control. In addition to these measures, some practices ask patients to complete standardized quality of life questionnaires. Expressed satisfaction with care is also a valid indicator of the impact of patient.

Standardized programs typically include specific evaluation criteria. To maintain reliability and validity, these tools cannot be altered.

ASTHMA EDUCATOR CERTIFICATION

Increasing costs of healthcare and managed care programs have placed pressure on the practitioner to manage clinic time efficiently. This situation has resulted in concern over having quality education time with patients. Reimbursement practices commonly drive the type of care delivered. At the time of this printing, asthma education is not reimbursable in many insurance plans, which means clinic time for such education may not be adequate in some practices. Specialty practices, where educators are certified, such as in diabetes practices, do receive reimbursement for patient education. In light of this, many certificate programs for asthma education are being offered by various groups. These programs are not regulated and do not measure outcomes.

The National Asthma Educator Certification Board (NAECB) was formed in 1999 and represents an interdisciplinary team of asthma experts to address the need for a standardized process for asthma certification. The goals of the NAECB are to standardize the certification process, evaluate the effectiveness of certified educators in disease management, and secure third party reimbursement for asthma education by counseling the Centers for Medicare and Medicaid Services. The first national certification examination was offered in 2002. Certification is a voluntary process, but some employers are requiring certification for certain positions. The NAECB Web site has information on the certification process. (www.naecb.org).

The Association of Asthma Educators (AAE) is an organization dedicated to raising the standard of asthma education and promoting consistency with national guidelines. The AAE offers a variety of educator workshops, including a review course for the national certification examination (www.asthmaeducators.org).

SUMMARY

Education is an essential component of asthma management. Despite clear guidelines, management goals are not meeting current national standards. Key asthma education concepts include the basic pathophysiology of asthma, the roles of medication, proper medication administration skills, environmental control measures, and when and how to respond to changes in asthma severity. Asthma education should be presented in a stepwise fashion.

A variety of teaching methods are appropriate to use, but no strategy replaces individual provider consultation with the patient and family. Effective asthma education is based on assessment of the learner, the theory of behavior change, cultural sensitivity, and evaluation of outcomes. Asthma education results in improved asthma control, decreased costs of healthcare, and patient and family satisfaction. The nurse is in an ideal position to advocate for the patient and family by providing asthma education that is consistent with national guidelines and tailored to individual needs.

CASE STUDY

Mrs. Garcia brings Juan, age 8, to the asthma clinic for the first time. The school nurse urged Mrs. Garcia to have Juan evaluated for asthma because he missed 21 days of school this year. He has had three ER visits and was released after "machine" treatments each time. Mrs. Garcia has been treating Juan with herbal tea, a soothing ointment that she applies to his chest, and rest for "congested breathing." She refuses to let Juan participate in physical education class or sports because he wheezes during strenuous activity. He awakens three times per week with a nocturnal cough. He also wakes up congested and wheezes when his dad smokes. Mr. Garcia wants Juan to play sports and insists that there is nothing wrong with his breath-

ing. The Garcia family has recently qualified for Medicaid.

Answer the following study questions, writing your responses on a separate sheet of paper. Compare your responses with the answers located at the end of the chapter.

1. What assessment issues should the nurse educator focus on for this visit?

2. What cultural assessments should the nurse complete?

3. What home therapies can safely be incorporated into the asthma management plan?

4. What are the priority teaching concepts for this visit?

5. What strategies can the nurse use to increase adherence to the treatment plan?

6. What can the nurse do to promote continued follow-up visits?

Answers to Case Study

1. The nurse should recognize that Mrs. Garcia could easily become overwhelmed with too much information. The focus should be on her and Juan's worries and concerns and the goals and expectations of treatment. Mrs. Garcia may have a fatalistic acceptance of Juan's ER visits, missed school days, and troublesome symptoms. It is important to raise her expectations. Juan should not miss school, have no ER visits, sleep through the night, and play sports without wheezing.

2. The nurse should assess who in the family influences decision-making. Mrs. Garcia did not take initiative in seeking care. She was directed to do so by the school nurse. Male figures and extended family tend to be important in Hispanic families. The father is certainly an important person to include in the management plan because it is indicated that he does not believe that his son has breathing difficulty and because he smokes. The mother or mother-in-

law may have passed down the tradition of home remedies and may influence Mrs. Garcia's decision to accept the treatment plan.

3. The herbal tea may be safe, but it would be best to assess the ingredients. It clearly does not replace asthma medication. The chest ointment is most likely safe. Rest is appropriate during an acute attack but is not appropriate as a routine practice.

4. The priority teaching concepts for this visit are to provide Mrs. Garcia and Juan with a basic understanding of asthma as a disease that does not go away, airway swelling, airway tightening, and the basic purpose and action of daily controller and quick-relief medications. They need to understand early warning signs of asthma exacerbations and to know when to call the provider for medical advice. This information needs to be kept at a basic level and reinforced and expanded at future visits.

5. The nurse can increase the likelihood of adherence by communicating interest and concern. The focus of the visit should be kept on priority issues and concerns for the family. A written treatment plan in the family's preferred language will increase adherence as will encouraging Mrs. Garcia to call if she has concerns.

6. The nurse can call to remind Mrs. Garcia of the next appointment. She can also request that Mrs. Garcia sign a consent for release of information so that the treatment plan can be shared with the school nurse. The school nurse has advocated for healthcare for Mrs. Garcia and she can be a valuable member of the team if she is included in communication.

EXAM QUESTIONS

CHAPTER 13
Questions 80-87

80. Asthma education begins when the

    a. diagnosis is made.

    b. family has accepted the chronic nature of asthma.

    c. patient has the first severe attack.

    d. patient returns for the second follow-up visit.

81. Findings from the U.S. Department of Health and Human Services Survey, Asthma Action America® indicate that

    a. there is a need for more effective patient education about asthma.

    b. patients grasp the basic concepts of asthma and its pathophysiology.

    c. levels of care currently meet national standards.

    d. most patients exhibit good asthma control.

82. The educational needs during the developmental stage of adolescence can best be met through

    a. self-directed learning.

    b. individual 1:1 counseling.

    c. support group with other teens.

    d. the Open Airways program.

83. Asthma education for the initial visit should include

    a. detailed information on trigger avoidance.

    b. patient fears related to asthma.

    c. evaluation of response to spirometry.

    d. information on immunotherapy.

84. Patients may be highly responsive to asthma education when they

    a. feel at ease.

    b. first learn of the diagnosis.

    c. have experienced a severe attack.

    d. are familiar with the asthma educator.

85. An advantage of videotaped instruction is that it

    a. effectively demonstrates skills such as inhaler technique.

    b. replaces the need for one-to-one education.

    c. is a substitute for written instruction.

    d. is easy to use in any setting.

86. To effectively evaluate clinical teaching the nurse must

    a. ask patients to complete knowledge surveys.

    b. assess patients for urgent care visits and activity tolerance.

    c. conduct follow-up telephone assessments.

    d. instruct the patient to keep a log of daily symptoms.

87. An advantage of obtaining asthma educator certification is that

    a. certification is always accompanied by a salary increase.

    b. the nurse can practice under her own established guidelines.

    c. the nurse has demonstrated competence in meeting national asthma education standards.

    d. patient satisfaction increases when taught by a certified nurse.

REFERENCES

Asthma in America. (2004). *Children and Asthma in America.* Retrieved December 21, 2004, from http://www.asthmainamerica.com/children _index.html

Brown, R., Bratton, S., Cabana, M., Kaciroti, N., & Clark, N. (2004). Physician asthma education program improves outcomes for children of low-income families. *Chest, 126*, 369-374.

Clark, N., Brown, R., Joseph, C., Anderson, E., Liu, M., & Valerio, M. (2004). Effects of a comprehensive school-based asthma program on symptoms, parent management, grades and absenteeism. *Chest, 125*, 1674-1679.

Doak, C., Doak, L., & Root, J. (1996). *Teaching patients with low literacy skills.* (2nd ed.) Philadelphia: J.B. Lippincott.

George, M. (2001). *Culturally-competent asthma education: A continuing education monograph.* Houston, TX: Association of Asthma Educators.

Gibson, P., Powell, H., Coughlan, J., Wilson, A., Abramson, M., Haywood, P., et al., (2002). *Self-management education and regular practitioner review for adults with asthma.* Retrieved December 8, 2004, from Cochrane Database of Systematic Reviews.

Janson, S., Fahy, J., Covington, J., Paul, S., Gold, W., & Boushey, H. (2003). Effects of individual self-management education on clinical, biological, and adherence outcomes in asthma. *American Journal of Medicine, 115*, 620-626.

Kyngäs, H. (2003). Patient education: Perspectives of adolescents with a chronic disease. *Journal of Clinical Nursing, 12,* 744-751.

Meng, A. & McConnell, S. (2003). Asthma education: Special applications for the school-age child. *Nursing Clinics of North America, 38,* 653-664.

National Asthma Education and Prevention Program. (1997). Expert panel report 2. *Guidelines for the diagnosis and management of asthma.* (NIH Publication No. 97-4051). Bethesda, MD: National Institutes of Health, National Heart, Lung, and Blood Institute. Available online at www.nhlbi.nih.gov/guidelines/asthma/index.pdf

National Heart, Lung, and Blood Institute/World Health Organization. (2003). *Global initiative for asthma: Global strategy for asthma management and prevention.* (NIH Publication No. 02-3659). Retrieved December 24, 2004, from http://www.ginasthma.com

Powell, H. & Gibson, P. (2002). Options for self-management education for adults with asthma. *The Cochrane Database of Systematic Reviews, 4.* Retrieved December 23, 2004, from http://gateway.ut.ovid.com/gw1/ovidweb.cgi

Rosenstock, I., Strecher, V., & Becker, M. (1988). Social learning theory and the health belief theory. *Health Education Quarterly, Summer, 15*(2), 175-183.

Wolf, F., Guevara, J., Grum, C., Clark, N., & Cates, C. (2002). *Educational interventions for asthma in children.* Retrieved December 23, 2004, from Cochrane Database of Systematic Reviews.

CHAPTER 14

WRITTEN ASTHMA SELF-MANAGEMENT PLANS

CHAPTER OBJECTIVE

Upon completion of this chapter, the reader will be able to recognize the role of written self-management plans in the overall plan of care and identify design characteristics that enhance the usefulness of these tools.

LEARNING OBJECTIVES

After studying this chapter, the reader will be able to

1. recognize the National Asthma Education and Prevention Program's (NAEPP's) recommendations on the use of written self-management guidelines.

2. identify controversies related to the use of written asthma self-management plans.

3. recognize three basic principles essential to effective self-management plans.

4. state the relationship of self-management plans to comprehensive asthma care.

5. identify five special planning needs for patients with asthma for trips away from home.

6. recognize patient input and modification to the plan as an essential aspect of partnership.

7. recognize the unique challenge of individualizing self-management plans for parents and children.

8. identify sources of recommended self-management plans.

OVERVIEW

The previous chapter discussed the central position of asthma education in comprehensive asthma management. Patient education is essential for achieving the best outcomes because of asthma's varying severity and the ongoing need for treatment adjustments at the earliest sign of deterioration. In responding early, patients and families must make decisions when healthcare consultation is not always available. The concept of written action plans arose when practitioners observed that delays in recognizing and treating exacerbations were contributing to poor asthma control. Written action plans summarize key education concepts in an individualized fashion for the patient and family. They serve as a guide to patient and family decision-making and are an essential component of asthma care.

NATIONAL ASTHMA EDUCATION AND PREVENTION PROGRAM RECOMMENDATIONS

The NAEPP recommends that written asthma action plans be included as an integral part of care. Written plans are especially important for patients with moderate or severe persistent asthma and for those patients with a history of severe exacerbations. Plans that guide day-to-day management of asthma, called "self-management plans," and "action plans," which guide responses to acute attacks, are recommended (NAEPP, 2003). Patients can receive self-management and action plans as two individual plans or they can be incorporated into one plan.

Many written plans are available. Recommended sources for written plans are included at the end of this chapter. Most plans divide action steps into three zones. The zone concept is identical to the peak flow zones with green representing asthma that is controlled, yellow representing beginning deterioration, and red representing danger or poor control. This concept is integrated into the written plan because it is based on a symbol that is easily recognized by all patients and families—the green, yellow, red traffic light.

However, not all patients need to monitor peak flow, and some patients are resistant to the recommendation to monitor peak flow readings on a daily basis or may not have the means to purchase a peak flow meter. Ideally, written plans allow flexibility for patients, such as linking treatment recommendations to severity of symptoms in addition to peak flow zones. The patient then has the option to select the preferred monitoring system.

The NAEPP recommends individualizing the nature and intensity of monitoring (2003). An example of individualizing the plan would be to identify the time of year that the person typically suffers the most asthma symptoms. In the case of the person who experiences an emergency room (ER) visit every October after the weather becomes cold, recommendations for monitoring could include logging symptoms on a diary or measuring peak flow twice-daily beginning in mid-September to determine the optimal time to begin or increase controller medication. During the spring and summer months, this patient can be given less intense monitoring recommendations.

Regardless of format used, the NAEPP recommends including specific content in the plan. These

recommendations are listed in Table 14-1. Clinicians should periodically review the plan, make revisions as needed, and confirm that the patient and family understands the plan. The family is advised to keep the plan in a handy location, such as on the refrigerator door, for easy reference. A copy of the plan is retained in the patient's medical record.

TABLE 14-1: NAEPP RECOMMENDATIONS FOR CONTENT TO BE INCLUDED ON WRITTEN SELF-MANAGEMENT PLANS

- Explicit, patient-specific recommendations for environmental control or other preventive measures

- A stepwise progression of procedures that clearly describes how to use controller and rescue medication

- Clear instructions on how to make medication adjustments when conditions change

- Steps the patient should take when medications are ineffective or if an emergency arises

- Provider contact information for securing urgent care

(NAEPP, 2002)

To be effective, the self-management plan must be imbedded in the total healthcare package (National Heart, Lung, and Blood Institute [NHLBI]/World Health Organization [WHO], 2003). It is fundamental to the plan that the patient recognizes early warning signs of deterioration of asthma control and seeks medical advice if there is no response to rescue medication or if nocturnal symptoms are experienced. Objective measuring, with either symptom diaries or peak flow recordings, are important because patients cannot reliably interpret subjective symptoms, especially those persons who have poor perception of airway obstruction.

Travel alters daily routines and access to usual healthcare resources. Patients and families commonly fail to consider asthma management in their trip plans. Special planning is required for trips away from home. The healthcare providers should initiate this discussion. See Table 14-2 for a list of travel plans.

TABLE 14-2: SELF-MANAGEMENT RECOMMENDATIONS FOR TRIPS AWAY FROM HOME

- Schedule a pre-trip visit with the healthcare provider.

- Obtain information about resources needed.

- Obtain a sufficient supply of medications.

- Determine availability of medications at the travel destination.

- Plan a system for memory aid during the nonroutine schedule period.

- Seek information in advance about availability of medical resources at the destination.

(NHLBI/WHO, 2003)

During pregnancy, the self-management plan should include prevention strategies to promote health of the infant after birth (NHLBI/WHO, 2003). Specific guidelines include the recommendation of breast-feeding as a measure for preventing infant asthma and allergy. Dust control if the mother has allergies to house dust mites and avoidance of active and passive smoking are essential content to include in the plan to reduce risk of asthma in the infant.

Some plans include a fourth zone, or action plan, which includes steps to follow in the event of an acute attack. Action plans include specific instructions for medication to be taken during an acute attack, including dose and frequency of dosing. Directions for assessment of symptoms as well as indications for seeking emergency care are listed. The action plan sometimes includes steps for initiating oral corticosteroids before seeking care in the ER. Recommendations for starting oral corticosteroids at home are based on the patient's history of rapid deterioration of asthma and the decision-making ability of the patient and family.

For pediatric patients, communicating treatment recommendations with the child's school is essential. Action plans for school include instructions not to send a child suspected of having an acute attack anywhere alone, indications for allowing the child to return to the classroom, instructions for when to call the parent, and the preferred hospital in the event that emergency care is needed. Ideally, the school plan is distributed to all adult school staff who would be in a position in which assessment of the child would be needed, including the bus driver and playground supervisor. Depending on state law, the school plan may indicate if the child's physician recommends that the child carry a rescue inhaler. Environmental triggers in the school environment that may predispose the child to an acute attack should also be identified.

CONTROVERSIES RELATED TO THE USE OF WRITTEN SELF-MANAGEMENT PLANS

Practitioner adherence to the use of written self-management plans is poor. As many as 50% to 70% of patients report never receiving a written plan from their provider, even through patients feel they would be useful. Numerous studies have been conducted to evaluate the impact of written plans on patient care outcomes. Unfortunately, a number of systematic reviews of randomized controlled trials conclude that the majority of these studies are methodologically flawed or lack sufficient power to draw any conclusions about the benefit of written plans (NAEPP, 2003; Lefevre et al., 2002; Toelle & Ram, 2004). Furthermore these studies lack sufficient evidence to determine if plans based on peak flow measurements or symptom-based plans improve care.

Evaluation of the impact of self-management plans is difficult because they are typically imbedded in the plan of care. It is not possible to isolate plans for study as the sole intervention in order to determine how they affect care outcomes. Therefore, when positive outcomes are evident, it is not possible to draw firm conclusions that the outcome was specifically related to the plan or to another aspect of the program intervention.

There is evidence of the effect of written plans from a nonrandomized case controlled study that used sound methodology. This study compared outcomes in patients who died from asthma to patients who presented to the hospital with an acute attack and survived. Patients who survived were more likely to have self-management plans. Written plans for patients with severe asthma were associated with a 70% reduction in risk for mortality (NAEPP, 2003).

Despite controversies regarding the benefit of plans, it is the position of the NAEPP that written self-management and action plans are an important component of care and that written plans improve patient-provider communication.

Readability of Written Plans

As noted above, there is poor compliance with written self-management plans in the United States. However, other countries have experienced improvements in day-to-day and acute care management with the use of written plans. A study using computerized software programs assessed the readability of seven national guideline plans and one international plan and compared these to plans developed in other countries (Forbis & Aligne, 2002). Self-management plans used in other countries were found to be simpler and easier to read.

The Forbis and Aligne study (2002) used findings from the National Adult Literacy Survey, which was conducted in 1993 to determine reading level of the U.S. population. Approximately 22% of the U.S. adult population is classified as functionally illiterate. Functional illiteracy correlates with a reading level of third grade or less. Another 25% to 28% of the U.S. population is classified as marginally illiterate, or reads below the fifth grade level. People at the lowest literacy levels are most likely to

be living in poverty and suffer higher rates and severity of asthma. In other words, the people in most need of written guidelines are least likely to be able to read them.

Self-management plans in the United States are generally written at the seventh to ninth grade levels. The most readable of the national or international plans reviewed was the Global Initiative for Asthma (NHLBI/WHO, 2003) plan. This plan was at a 5.7 grade reading level. Systematic computer programs are not available to assess other components of written plans, but characteristics such as use of color, active voice, common words, short sentences, and visual cues enhance comprehension. Most of the United States plans also rated poor in regard to these characteristics.

Some patients will not be able to read any plan, even if readability is judged as acceptable. Written plans are still recommended for these patients because they can be used to enhance communication with other care providers. Color coding or visual cues are especially helpful in these cases. In the author's experience, patients who have a difficult time reading have been able to follow plans that used a system of color-coded dots. For example, patients with poor reading skills were taught to match a blue dot placed on the bottom of the canister of rescue medication to the blue dot on the management plan that indicated the frequency and number of puffs of rescue medication to use. A different color was used to match the inhaled corticosteroid canister to corticosteroid dosing instructions on the written plan.

Unintended messages may be imbedded in written plans. When the majority of space on written plans is devoted to the management of acute attacks, patients assume that attack management is the most important factor (Milnes & Callery, 2003). In this case, patients may downplay the importance of every day control measures. Priority issues should be spatially balanced on written plans.

Two plans written by practitioners in Rochester, New York were evaluated as most readable, that is at the 4.9 and 5.9 grade levels (Forbis & Aligne, 2002). The Rochester Regional Community Asthma Network developed the Finger Lakes Asthma Action Plan which is illustrated in Figure 14-1. This plan uses a three-zone concept and incorporates color, common words, visual cues with the option of symptom-based or peak flow–based assessment methods. A Spanish translation and directions for healthcare providers are also available. See Figure 14-2 for the directions for the healthcare provider.

SELF-MANAGEMENT PLANS AND PEDIATRIC APPLICATIONS

Between the ages of 7 and 17, parents' assessments of children's asthma symptoms and perceptions of quality of life do not correlate (Milnes & Callery, 2003). Parents consistently underestimate children's symptoms. The theory of illness perception is based on the assumption that interpretation of symptoms is not made by one individual for another, but is a personal, subjective assessment. Clinical practice with respect to the use of self-management plans for children is not consistent with illness perception theory because the concept of "good" control differs between parents and children.

Parents tend to interpret asthma as tolerable if the child is free from acute attacks. Children, on the other hand, give more evidence to how asthma affects their daily lives. Healthcare providers may have even different expectations from parents and children. Effective use of self-management plans requires that expectations between all parties are clear and that all parties participate in goal setting.

Concepts and language on self-management plans do not necessarily mean the same thing to parents and children. Survey responses from 47 asthma centers indicated that practitioners feel there is a need for developmentally based management plans for children that include increased flexibility for decision-making (Milnes & Callery, 2003). Roles for parents and children need to be clarified. Vague language such as "if your asthma gets worse, do this" provides little guidance for assessment and intervention. Perhaps children's asthma plans should be based on interference with activities of daily living and play, with indications for actions the child should take and indications for when to tell an adult about early warning signals.

An asthma action plan for infants and young children is available (Figure 14-3) (Wakefield, 2004). This plan incorporates symptom monitoring because young children are developmentally incapable of performing peak flow maneuvers. Clear delineation of asthma symptoms using color codes, and a basic physical assessment guide to indicators of respiratory distress in infants and young children are strengths of this action plan. Parents become very anxious when young children experience breathing difficulty and should benefit from the chart that classifies wheezing in terms parents can understand. Normal respiratory rates are included, as well as specific indications for calling the healthcare provider.

Computerized plans lend themselves to individualization. Adolescents have critiqued asthma education because it fails to use computer technology. Participation in designing individualized computer-based plans may appeal to adolescents.

PARTNERSHIP IN PLANNING

The NAEPP (2003) emphasizes that partnership in care is as important as assessment, environmental control, and medical management. Partnership means shared decision-making regarding therapeutic goals and options. Involvement of patients and families in the development of individ-

(text continues on page 186)

FIGURE 14-1: ROCHESTER REGIONAL COMMUNITY ASTHMA NETWORK: THE FINGER LAKES ASTHMA ACTION PLAN

Finger Lakes Asthma Action Plan

(To Be Completed By Health Care Provider)

Updated On: _____

Name: _____ Date of Birth: _____ Grade____ Address: _____

School Year: 200__ -- 200__   School/Daycare: _____   Emergency Contact/Phone: _____

Asthma Severity   ☐ Mild Intermittent   ☐ Mild Persistent   ☐ Moderate Persistent   ☐ Severe Persistent

Asthma Triggers   ☐ Colds   ☐ Exercise   ☐ Animals   ☐ Dust   ☐ Smoke   ☐ Food   ☐ Weather   ☐ Other

1. Green Zone: Good Control

Child feels good:
- Breathing is good
- No cough or wheeze
- Can work/play
- Sleeps all night

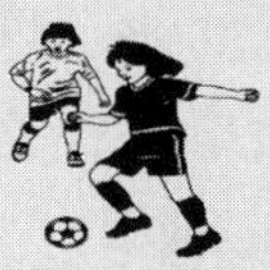

Personal Best Peak Flow_____

Peak flow in this area most of time:
_____ to_____

Controller Medicine - Use Every Day

Controller Medicine (Take At Home)	How much	When to take it

20 minutes before sports use this medicine:
_____

Student may carry and use this medicine at school. (Check box)
☐ YES   ☐ NO

2. Yellow Zone: Be Careful

Child has any of these:
- Cough
- Wheeze
- Tight Chest
- Wakes up at night

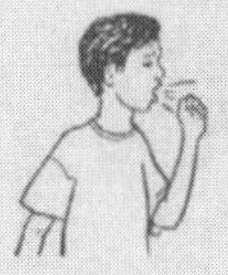

Peak flow in this area most of time:
_____ to_____

Take Daily Controller Medicine in Green Zone and Add this Reliever Medicine when needed for an asthma episode

Reliever Medicine	How much	When to take it

Student may carry and use this medicine at school. (Check box)
☐ YES   ☐ NO

Call doctor if these medicines are used more than two times a week in the day or two times a month at night.

3. Red Zone: DANGER CALL DOCTOR NOW!

Child has any of these:
- Medicine not helping
- Breathing hard & fast
- Nose opens wide
- Can't walk or talk well
- Ribs show

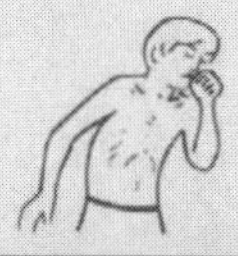

Peak flow below:

Take These Medicines

Medicine	How much	When to take it

911 Lips are bluish, Getting worse fast, Struggling to breathe, Can't talk/cry because of hard breathing or Has passed out

Health Care Provider Name: _____ Phone:_____ Fax:_____

Health Care Provider Signature: _____ Date: _____

Patient/Parent Signature: _____ Date: _____

WHITE – PATIENT COPY   YELLOW – SCHOOL/DAY CARE COPY   PINK – PROVIDER COPY

Developed by the Regional Community Asthma Network of the Finger Lakes (RCAN) and adapted from NHLBI - 9/01 revised 3/04

Note. Action Plan reproduced with permission of Regional Community Asthma Network of the Finger Lakes: www.rcanasthma.net

**FIGURE 14-2: ROCHESTER REGIONAL COMMUNITY ASTHMA NETWORK
THE FINGER LAKES ASTHMA ACTION PLAN
DIRECTIONS TO HEALTH CARE PROVIDERS**

Directions to the Health Care Provider
In Completing this Asthma Action Plan For Schools and Daycares

This plan is designed to help children and families improve control of their asthma and provide instructions in the event of an exacerbation at school. The patient /family should be able to demonstrate that they understand how to use this plan, and the medications you have prescribed.

- This form has been designed for the primary care provider to use with families who need a relatively simple asthma management regimen.
- Once a family has become more informed about asthma, a plan can be developed with additional flexibility in treatment.
- Families should be given additional educational materials about asthma, peak flow monitoring, and environmental control.

When completing the plan:

- **Do not** use medical abbreviations such as bid, PO or q4. Please use twice a day, by mouth or every 4 hours.
- Check off the patient's asthma severity level and triggers that may cause symptoms.
- Sign the form and fill in your office phone and fax number.
- Have the parent sign the asthma action plan.
- Give the White copy to the family/patient, the Yellow copy to the school/day care center and keep the Pink copy for your records. THE YELLOW COPY IS THE ONLY FORM THAT SHOULD BE PROVIDED TO THE SCHOOL!

Complete information for each zone as follows.

- Green Zone:
  Please list all controller medicines the patient takes on a **DAILY** basis.
  How much and how often to take them.
  Identify reliever medicine the patient should use before PE/Sports/Exercise.
  Mark YES when you and the parent want their child to **CARRY & USE** medicine at school.
- Yellow Zone:
  Please add any reliever/rescue medications that should be taken.
  Instruct the patient to continue with green zone medicines.
  Include how long to continue taking these medicines and when to contact the provider.

- Red Zone:
  Explain to the patient that these symptoms indicate an asthma emergency.
  List any medications to be taken while waiting to speak to the provider or preparing to go to the emergency room.

- Peak flow readings are **optional** but do help school health care providers and parents to assess severity of symptoms and effectiveness of medication.
  - The "Personal Best" peak flow should be determined when the child is symptom-free. A diary can be used to determine personal best, and usually are part of the peak flow meter package.
  - A peak flow reading should be taken at all asthma visits and personal best should be redetermined regularly. Because peak flow readings may vary with the meter used instruct your patients to bring their peak flow meter to every visit.

This action plan was developed by the Regional Community Asthma Network of the Finger Lakes (RCAN) and adapted from the National Heart, Lung and Blood Institute. If there are any questions or you require more plans, please feel free to call (585) 442-4260.

Revised 3/04

Note. Action Plan reproduced with permission of Regional Community Asthma Network of the Finger Lakes: www.rcanasthma.net

FIGURE 14-3: ASTHMA ACTION PLAN FOR INFANTS AND YOUNG CHILDREN (1 OF 2)

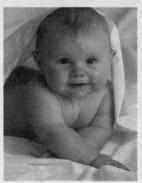

Asthma Action Plan for Infants and Young Children

Child's Name:_____

Date:_____

Doctor:_____

Phone for Doctor:_____

Green Zone—All Clear
Your baby or young child feels good, sleeps without symptoms, eats without trouble, and acts normal.

Use control medicine every day

_____

_____

Yellow Zone—Caution
Your child is having a flare-up: mild coughing, wheezing or whistling in chest, shortness of breath. Symptoms cause trouble with usual activities or sleeping. *Important: if symptoms continue for 12-24 hrs—call the doctor.*

Take quick relief medicine* when there is a flare-up. *Important: keep taking control medicine daily.*

_____

_____

*If your child needs quick relief medicine more than 2-3 times/week, call the doctor.

Red Zone—Danger, Medical Alert!
This is an **emergency**—get help! Symptoms are: rapid breathing, feeding stops, crying is softer/ shorter, nostrils open wider, grunting sound during feeding, skin pale or red in the face, wheezing or whistling in chest increases, skin between ribs is pulled tight.

Give Quick-Relief Medicine right away and get help from the doctor or call 911 now!

_____

_____

_____

FIGURE 14-3: ASTHMA ACTION PLAN FOR INFANTS AND YOUNG CHILDREN (2 OF 2)

Call the Doctor Right Away for Any of These Symptoms in Your Child

- *If your child has a history of having to go to the Emergency Room or being hospitalized for breathing problems in the past, call the doctor* **early***, before wheeze, cough, or shortness of breath gets worse*
- Infants: Trouble feeding; shorter, softer cry; difficulty laying down due to trouble breathing
- Toddlers: Difficulty talking, walking, or playing because of trouble breathing.
- Mild to moderate wheezing, coughing, or shortness of breath for **12 to 24 hours** and not relieved by medication.
- Rapidly increasing shortness of breath, or difficulty breathing.
- Strained neck muscles when breathing.
- When child is breathing, the skin sinks in between the ribs or at the base of the throat (retractions).
- Tiredness due breathing trouble.
- Wheezing when breathing in as well as breathing out.
- Lips and tongue turning blue; gasping for air (**call 911**).

Stop, Look and Listen:
Things to Tell the Doctor

Child's Current Condition:
Breathing Rate while *sleeping*: ___ breaths per minute

□ Breathing *in* takes longer than normal
□ Breathing *out* takes longer than normal

Color of skin, tongue and lips: _____

Wheeze:	Yes □	No □
Retractions:	Yes □	No □
Tiredness:	Yes □	No □

When did symptoms begin? _____
Was child exposed to possible trigger? _____
If yes, what trigger? _____

What I Did to Help My Child:
Medications:
   Name: _____
   Dose: _____
   How often: _____
   How long ago: _____
Other things I did: _____
Did the symptoms:
   □ Get Better   □ Stay the same
   □ Get Worse

Normal *Sleeping* Breathing Rates for Infants and Young Children

Child's Age	Breathing Rate (Breaths/Minute)
1-3 months old	35-55
3-6 months old	30-45
6-12 months old	25-40
1-3 years old	20-30
3-6 years old	20-25

How Bad is the Wheezing?

Mild: Child wheezes only on breathing out.

Moderate: Wheezes with breathing in or breathing out.

Severe: There may be no wheezing at all due to *severe* trouble breathing.

Note. Used with permission. Developed by Peggy L. Wakefield, MD, FAAP, for the Peer to Peer HealthCare Provider Asthma Education Program. Copyright Peggy L. Wakefield and the Coastal Bend Health Education Center, an affiliate of the Texas A&M University System Health Science Center, 2004.

ualized self-management plans is an ideal situation for fostering partnership in asthma care.

A criticism of many available plans is that they are a set of instructions to be followed. Self-management plans are becoming unpopular with healthcare providers and patients, even though patients indicated the need for some type of written management guides. One theory suggests that written plans are difficult to use because they are derived from the medical perspective rather than the patient perspective (Douglass et al., 2002). An interview study was conducted with adults with asthma to validate this explanation. Patients who used their plans modified them based on their personal experience with symptoms. For instance, a plan may direct a patient to go to the ER if the peak flow reading is 50% below the individual's personal best. This patient may have the experience of deteriorating rapidly. Waiting until the peak flow reaches 50% of best may be too late an indicator. This patient should modify his plan to go to the ER when his peak flow is at 65% of personal best. (Optimally, controller medication in appropriate doses is taken consistently so that peak flow does not drop dangerously low.) This type of knowledge only comes from the personal experience of living with asthma. Ideally, patients should have the flexibility to make this type of decision.

Interestingly, denial about diagnosis was not a barrier to consulting the plan. In fact, patients who were not given a plan by their provider sometimes created their own plan (Douglass et al., 2002). Most patients found that plans were useful to them, but interpretation of the plan from a personal perspective of experience with asthma is vital to implementation. Clinicians should expect patients to modify their plans and inquire about modifications in follow up visits.

THE NURSE'S ROLE IN SELF-MANAGEMENT PLANS

As discussed in chapter 13, the nurse is in an ideal position to provide education because he or she is perceived as approachable and often has time to spend with patients and families. Time spent with families should include discussion of the self-management plan.

Depending on the practice, the primary provider or the nurse may be accountable for writing the plan. The plan is always based on the primary provider's treatment recommendations, regardless of who completes the plan. Goals of therapy should be incorporated into the plan. Adherence increases when patients and families are involved in setting treatment goals. Patients should be asked, "What do you want to be able to do that you cannot do now?" The patient's response, such as wanting to make the track team, play the horn, or even sleep through the night, can be written on the plan.

Patient preference for symptom or peak flow monitoring can be taken into account. However, there may be times when the patient needs to be encouraged to monitor peak flow readings. To illustrate, a 12-year-old patient should be able to independently recognize early warning signs. A 12-year-old patient presented to the clinic giving a history of approaching other students in the class and asking them if they thought she was having difficulty breathing. She based her decision to use rescue medication on their input. The other students had no physical assessment skills or knowledge of asthma. The nurse focused discussion on the signals the child was using to determine her need to consult the other students. The parent and child agreed that she was aware of some breathing signals but lacked confidence to label them herself. They agreed that recognition of symptoms was the child's responsibility and that use of the peak flow meter would validate her impressions and help build decision-making confidence. In this case, the patient and family were directed toward the choice to use peak flow meters, and they participated in that decision.

Patients and families can participate in medication-related decisions. Assuming the patient can perform administration maneuvers correctly, adherence improves if the patient's preference for metered-dose inhaler or dry powered inhaler is considered. Timing of controller medication dosing should also be incorporated into the patient's plan. Patients typically prefer linking dosing to a routine activity, such as brushing their teeth in the morning and evening. Patients who are taking multiple doses of a low-strength corticosteroid may appreciate learning that dosing can be less frequent with a higher concentration of the medication. They will commonly make the decision to purchase the higher concentration formulation.

The initial plan should be kept as simple as possible and should include specific instructions for when to call for advice. Examples of specific instructions are, "if you start taking your rescue medication more than twice per week call the clinic" or, "if your peak flow readings fall to 225 for two days in a row call the clinic." Patients should be asked on subsequent clinic visits if they used their plan and if they made modifications. Patients and families should participate in revisions to the plan.

RECOMMENDED SOURCES OF SELF-MANAGEMENT PLANS

The NAEPP has self-management plans and student action plans that are designed for use in schools. These plans can be downloaded from the National Heart, Lung, and Blood Institute's Web site: (www.nhlbi.nih.gov/health/prof/lung/asthma).

The NAEPP plans are between seventh- to ninth-grade reading levels and may be best adapted for use in private practices.

The American Lung Association has self-management plans in English and Spanish. They incorporate use of color but do not include visual cues. Visit www.lungusa.org to download these forms.

The Global Initiative for Asthma (GINA) has a link on their Web site, www.ginasthma.org, to patient and family resources. The patient and family resources contain basic information about asthma in simple terms and include a simple self-management plan. GINA also has self-management forms with color and visual cues available from the National Institutes of Health. The publication number is 96-3659C. The email address is nihinfo@OD.NIH.gov

The Rochester Regional Community Asthma Network developed the self-management plan evaluated as most readable. This plan, entitled Finger Lakes Asthma Action Plan, can be downloaded at http://www.rcanasthma.net. The Spanish version can also be downloaded from this Web site as well as directions for professionals on the use of the self-management plans.

The nurse may wish to explore self-management plans that are available locally, especially through state or local asthma coalitions. Local plans may be useful if language has been adapted to the unique characteristics of the local population. The nurse can evaluate self-management plans using the criteria discussed above in the section entitled "Readability of Written Plans."

SUMMARY

Written asthma self-management plans are an integral component of asthma care. Attempts to study the individual impact of written plans on asthma outcomes have been flawed by methodological problems, but use of written plans has been associated with decreased asthma mortality. The NAEPP strongly endorses the use of individualized written plans developed in partnership with patients and families. Plans should link treatment decisions to peak flow or symptom assessments. The most effective plans are written at a fifth grade reading level, enhance communication with color and visual cues, and allow for flexible patient decision-making. Management plans for parents and children need to clarify roles of family members and what is meant by "good" control. Nurses can increase adherence by incorporating the patient's and the family's goals and treatment preferences on the written plan.

CASE STUDY

Mrs. Mitchell comes to the asthma clinic with her 4-year-old granddaughter, Mary. Mrs. Mitchell is Mary's primary caretaker and sole breadwinner in the family. She is frustrated because Mary's Headstart program calls once or twice per week asking her to take Mary home because of wheezing. When this occurs, Mrs. Mitchell treats Mary with albuterol via nebulizer around the clock for 24 hours and then sends her back to school. She is tired of waking up for the overnight treatments but states, "that's just the way it has to be."

Mary is evaluated as having moderate persistent asthma and is started on budesonide 0.5 mg via nebulizer three times daily.

Answer the following study questions, writing your responses on a separate sheet of paper. Compare your responses with the answers located at the end of the chapter.

1. How can the nurse direct Mrs. Mitchell's frustrations with frequent calls from the school and nocturnal awakenings toward setting therapeutic goals?

2. What indications for the use of albuterol should the nurse incorporate on the written self-management plan?

3. What medication delivery device should the nurse introduce to Mrs. Mitchell?

4. How should Mrs. Mitchell monitor Mary's symptoms?

5. What communication should occur with Mary's school?

6. What comprehension cues will most likely increase Mrs. Mitchell's use of the written plan?

Answers to Case Study

1. Empathetic statements from the nurse would indicate understanding of Mrs. Mitchell's stress related to Mary's poor asthma control. Mrs. Mitchell's response that "its just the way it has to be" is fatalistic. She does not perceive the ability to change the course of events. The nurse should clearly explain that Mary's symptoms are mostly preventable. Clarify with Mrs. Mitchell that she seems most upset with the night awakenings and calls from school. When agreement is reached, write these two issues as the primary goals on the plan. The plan will read, "Mary will remain in school every day with no wheezing," and "Mary will sleep through every night with no cough."

2. Mrs. Mitchell is relying on albuterol as the sole asthma medication. Her use of albuterol is excessive. She needs to clearly understand the role of controller medication and to expect that, when given every day, it is effective in preventing symptoms. The plan should clearly state to administer albuterol only when acute symptoms are present and to call the healthcare provider if it is used more than twice per week.

3. Medication delivery is more accurate and convenient when administered via metered-dose (MDI) inhaler and spacer than with the nebulizer. Because Mary is 4-years-old, she would benefit from a spacer with facemask. The portability and short administration time will most likely appeal to Mrs. Mitchell, but it requires more active participation from Mary than the nebulizer treatments. Demonstration and return demonstration need to be given. The

nurse should carefully assess Mrs. Mitchell's and Mary's ability with the device. The nurse will need to consult with the provider to change the medication prescription to fluticasone because budesonide is not available in inhaler form. Mrs. Mitchell may need to be instructed to practice the MDI technique with Mary before complete changeover is accomplished.

4. Mary is too young for a peak flow meter; therefore, symptom monitoring is the assessment method of choice. The nurse should carefully review signs of respiratory distress with Mrs. Mitchell, including counting respirations and observing for nasal flaring and retracting. She should note the frequency of nocturnal awakenings and understand that this is a sign that Mary's asthma is out of control.

5. It would appear that the school has no action plan for Mary and that they have no rescue medication on hand. This assumption needs to be validated with Mrs. Mitchell. Assess the preschool's policy about administering medication. Give Mrs. Mitchell a copy of the written plan to send to the preschool. If school policy permits administration of medication, a signed permission note from the physician needs to be sent to the school.

6. The plan needs to be simple and should use common words, color, and visual cues. Words such as "wakes up at night" should be substituted for "nocturnal asthma." Green, yellow, and red colors highlighting severity levels of symptoms help distinguish level of asthma control. Visual cues such as pictures of a child actively playing, coughing, or in distress also aid understanding. Confirm that Mrs. Mitchell has the telephone number of the provider and emphasize that she can call in the middle of the night for help with decision-making.

EXAM QUESTIONS

CHAPTER 14
Questions 88-92

88. According to the NAEPP, principles incorporated into self-management plans should include

    a. flexible recommendations for environmental control.

    b. a fixed list of medication dosages to use.

    c. steps the patient should take when medications are ineffective.

    d. health insurance benefit information.

89. The best self-management plans contain

    a. long complete sentences.

    b. medical terms, not lay terms.

    c. color and visual cues.

    d. passive voice.

90. Recommendations for planning trips away from home include

    a. developing a plan to remember to take medications.

    b. after arriving at the destination, seek out potential sources of medical advice.

    c. increasing controller medication prior to the trip in the event of exposure to unknown triggers.

    d. scheduling a post-trip visit with the provider.

91. Parents' interpretation of their child's asthma symptoms

    a. are accurate by either parent or child because they tend to agree about the severity of symptoms.

    b. is always different than the interpretation by the child.

    c. is consistently an underestimated interpretation.

    d. is usually an over-reactive interpretation.

92. In terms of flexibility, the most effective self-management plans

    a. allow for decision-making based on the patient's experience with asthma.

    b. provide a clear list of explicit instructions.

    c. are developed from tested medical points of view.

    d. are modified by the primary provider only.

REFERENCES

Douglass, J., Aroni, R., Goeman, D., Stewart, K., Sawyer, S., Thien, F., & Abramson, M. (2002). A qualitative study of action plans for asthma. *British Medical Journal, 324*, 1-5.

Forbis, S. & Aligne, A. (2002). Poor readability of written asthma management plans found in national guidelines. *Pediatrics, 109*(4), Retrieved October 10, 2004, from http://www.pediatrics.org

Lefevre, F., Piper, M., Weiss, K., Mark, D., Clark, N. & Aronson, N. (2002). Do written action plans improve patient outcomes in asthma? An evidenced-based analysis. *Journal of Family Practice, 51*(19), 842-848.

Milnes, L. & Callery, P. (2003). The adaptation of written self-management plans for children with asthma. *Issues and Innovations in Nursing Practice, 41*(5), 444-453.

National Asthma Education and Prevention Program. (2003). Expert Panel Report: *Guidelines for the diagnosis and management of asthma: Update on selected topics 2002.* (NIH Publication No. 02-5074). Bethesda, MD: National Institutes of Health, National Heart, Lung and Blood Institute. Available online at http://www.nhlbi.nih.gov/guidelines/asthma/index.html

National Heart, Lung, and Blood Institute/World Health Organization. (2003). *Global initiative for asthma: Global strategy for asthma management and prevention.* (NIH Publication No. 02-3659). Retrieved December 24, 2004, from http://www.ginasthma.com

Toelle, B. & Ram, F. (2004). *Written individualized management plans for asthma in children and adults.* Retrieved October 10, 2004, from Cochrane Database of Systematic Reviews.

Wakefield, P. (2004). For the Peer to Peer HealthCare Provider Asthma Education Program. *Asthma action plan for infants and young children.* Corpus Christi, TX.

CHAPTER 15

ASTHMA CAMP—A UNIQUE EDUCATIONAL OPPORTUNITY FOR CHILDREN AND FAMILIES

CHAPTER OBJECTIVE

Upon completion of this chapter, the reader will be able to recognize unique benefits of asthma education in the camp setting for children with asthma and their parents.

LEARNING OBJECTIVES

After studying this chapter, the reader will be able to

1. identify five characteristics of an effective asthma camp program.

2. identify children who would benefit most from an asthma camp program.

3. recognize five teaching and learning principles that promote learning in a group setting.

4. recognize sports participation as a learning opportunity for the child with asthma.

5. recognize the impact of creative learning strategies on child and parent learning.

6. identify two methods of individualizing education in a camp setting.

7. recognize why evaluation of camp program outcomes is a priority.

8. state two ways that camp programs impact community relationships and interdisciplinary teamwork.

9. identify two ways that nurses in clinical practice can support children attending asthma camps.

OVERVIEW

Asthma camps provide a unique opportunity to provide children with developmentally based asthma education. Nurses should be informed of the benefits of camp programs so they can provide up-to-date information to children with asthma and their families. This chapter describes a children's asthma day camp and lessons learned from camp experiences over an 11-year period. Camps for children are labor intensive but provide a unique opportunity to enhance asthma education for children in creative and exciting ways.

This chapter describes the development of an educational asthma camp program from the design of a mission statement and underlying theoretical frameworks to program outcome evaluation. This particular program has brought a high degree of satisfaction to the children, families, interdisciplinary team, students, and academic community that it has touched. It is hoped that the ideas presented in this chapter will stimulate the reader to design creative asthma education interventions for children and families in their care.

CHARACTERISTICS OF EFFECTIVE ASTHMA CAMP PROGRAMS

Clear Purpose

Children with asthma commonly do not meet the health requirements of regular summer camps. Many camps designed specifically for children with asthma are intended only to provide the child with a happy camping experience because they are not eligible for regular camps. This is a valid purpose to design an asthma camp; however, the intended purpose drives program planning and content. Many of these camps lack a strong educational component because the primary goal is camping.

Camp Reactive Airway Disease (RAD) was created to find a solution to the high rates of hospitalization and lack of asthma education among children with asthma. Other less labor-intensive educational strategies were explored before developing the camp program. These strategies included hospital-based education, parent education programs with flexible hours to meet scheduling needs of working parents, programming enticements such as offering food, and physician recommendations. These methods were ineffective. Hospitalized children were not receptive to comprehensive education because of the acute effects of asthma. Parents were resistant to returning to the hospital for educational programs. Program enticements had no effect. As a result of these experiences, the focus of program planning changed. A different purpose was developed to design a program to provide preventive asthma education directly to school-age children in a way that was fun. A secondary purpose was to indirectly impact parent learning through the child.

Mission Statement

Planning started with development of a mission statement. This step is critical because clear mission statements define beliefs and values about the nature of the program. These beliefs serve as a guide to program planning and future program revisions and help communicate the intent of the program to others. Critical values included in the Camp RAD mission statement are listed in Table 15-1.

TABLE 15-1: CRITICAL VALUES AS DESCRIBED IN THE CAMP RAD MISSION STATEMENT

- The purpose of camp is to provide asthma education.
- Asthma education is based on sound learning, cognitive, and developmental theories.
- Parents are essential partners in managing the child's asthma.
- Asthma education is consistent with the National Asthma Education and Prevention Program Guidelines.
- Children should be able to participate in physical activities to the fullest extent possible.
- Learning is enhanced when it is fun.
- Interdisciplinary teamwork enhances program development.
- Evaluation is a critical component of the program.

To illustrate usefulness of the mission statement, Camp RAD was designed as a local day camp rather than a residential camp because the team held the belief that parents are important partners in care. Day programs facilitate parental contact because parents are required to transport the child to and from camp each day. Also, the local nature of the camp allowed for a program for parents to be incorporated into the last day's agenda. An unforeseen benefit was that children with asthma who were anxious about leaving home were more receptive to a day program than a residential out-of-town program. Typically, these were the children who were most in need of asthma education.

The mission statement has served the Camp RAD program well. Suggestions from parents or team members to alter the program are examined from the perspective of program values. Suggestions that are compatible with the program's purpose and values are incorporated into the program. If suggestions lack consistency with the mission statement, clearly written values help explain programming decisions.

Evidenced-Based Guidelines as Part of Program Design

The National Asthma Education and Prevention Program (NAEPP) (NAEPP, 1997; NAEPP, 2003) provides the most complete consensus of asthma experts on the diagnosis and management of asthma. The NAEPP guidelines direct the healthcare delivered by the asthma camp team and are essential to the development of the children's asthma camp curriculum. Asthma health education topics include basic understanding of asthma, symptom monitoring, early warning sign recognition, trigger avoidance, medications, and exercise-induced asthma prevention. These topics are consistent with NAEPP recommendations for goals of care and health education. The NAEPP guidelines are also the foundation of the instructional content in counselor training workshops.

Foundational Theories of Program Design

Effective programs are theory-based. Theories that explain personality and cognitive development and how children learn are foundational to the Camp RAD program.

Erik Erikson's (1963) psychosocial theory of personality development explains the major task of the school-age child as resolving the conflict between industry and inferiority. The stage of industry is characterized by mastery of new tasks and skills, striving to meet the expectations of others, conforming to avoid disapproval, and a desire for success that is rewarded. Successful completion of these tasks leads to a sense of self-esteem.

Erikson's psychosocial theory is applied to the camp program in several ways. For example, new skills, such as use of peak flow meters, are introduced in small groups with instruction on a level consistent with the child's cognitive ability. Skills are introduced in small steps and demonstrated to ensure mastery. Individual reinforcement and praise are imbedded throughout camp activities. Because children strive to meet expectations of others, expectations of the camp staff for campers are clearly articulated at the beginning of the program and continually reinforced. The grand program finale rewards success with an awards ceremony at which each child is recognized for skills achieved in both asthma management and general camp activities.

Piaget's theory of cognitive development (1969) provides a framework for the camp asthma education program. According to Piaget, the school- age child's thinking is characterized by concrete operations. Distinctive aspects of this theory that guide the camp plan are: school-age children are systematic and logical thinkers; they have longer attention spans than in the preschool years; they can deal with multiple aspects of a situation at one time; they understand time, space and rules; and they can appreciate different points of view but cannot think abstractly. Motion, action, and multisensory teaching approaches enhance the school-age child's learning.

The camp asthma curriculum is designed to progress logically and systematically from a basic understanding of the parts of the airway to characteristics of the healthy airway to airway changes during an acute attack and, eventually, to how quick-relief and long term controller medications work in the airway. Children's cognitive appreciation of space allows for instruction to focus on the impact of swelling on airway space available for breathing. Campers understand quick-relief and long-term controller actions because they have a cognitive understanding of time. They are also able to appreciate early versus late warning signs. The ability to understand different points of view allows for discussion of various trigger avoidance and relaxation strategies. Classes are designed with as many visual, tactile and motion strategies as possible. For instance, the medication class includes personification of rescue and controller inhalers. Children role-play a constricted bronchiole as others race to the rescue with quick-acting inhalers.

By far the most challenging content to teach is the concept of airway swelling because it is an abstract concept. School-age children lack the ability to think abstractly. The teaching model, Radical Randy,™ was designed to fill this educational gap. (See chapter 14 for a description of the model.) The three-dimensional character of the model allows children to visualize swelling and see the narrowing of the airway. In other words, the model makes an abstract concept concrete, thus educational content remains consistent with cognitive developmental theory.

Professional Nature of Staff

Camp is a creative approach to offering healthcare, but planning must incorporate traditional standards of care. Although the camp setting is informal, staff members are bound by the same professional duty to the patient and family that exists in the clinic or acute care environment. Camp staff must understand professional ethics, confidentiality, and legal implications of care. They must be grounded in theory and knowledge of pediatrics and specialty asthma concepts. Camp represents a contractual agreement with the patient and family. Staff are accountable for maintaining a high level of professional standards.

Given the nature of the camp program as a healthcare setting, professional background in one of the healthcare fields (nursing, medicine, respiratory therapy, pharmacy, etc.) is a requirement of all staff who assume direct responsibility for care of the campers. An interdisciplinary pediatric asthma team

serves as core camp planners and managers. The team includes a pediatric nurse practitioner, pediatric allergy-immunologist, respiratory therapist, health educator, and a child life specialist. Each year a new group of counselors is recruited from university health professions schools. Students include nursing, medical, and respiratory therapy students. All students have completed several semesters of school and have an understanding of professional ethics and basics of patient and family care. Given these attributes, students are then recruited based on their love of working with children and families.

Staff Training

Counselors participate in 3 days of intensive camp workshops. During the workshop, 8 hours are devoted to asthma specialty content, 8 hours are spent reviewing camp-specific policies and activity management, and the remaining 8 hours focus on mastery of the asthma teaching content. Educational theory and principles of learning are integrated into the counselor classes on teaching. Counselors apply these principles as they teach the asthma camp classes to the children. They receive academic course credit for their work.

CHARACTERISTICS OF CHILDREN LIKELY TO BENEFIT FROM ASTHMA CAMP

Camp is a labor-intensive project. Due to the intensity of the project, it is costly. Estimated cost per camper is $1,500.00. This is a significant investment in each child and places responsibility on program planners to ensure that intended outcomes are achieved. Outcomes are dependent, in part, on ensuring that children in need of asthma education attend the program. Children must also be capable of learning the content.

Children most in need of asthma education are those with persistent forms of asthma. The program is offered in English, so campers must be English-speaking. Campers must also be between ages 7 and 12. Six year olds were accepted in the first camp session but were unable to process the asthma content and lacked endurance for planned camping activities. Seven year olds have sufficient developmental maturity to participate but asthma sessions are taught at a more basic level for the younger children. Adolescents are capable of understanding content, but planning would require significant modifications suited to their unique developmental needs.

Some children with asthma have comorbid illnesses such as diabetes or sickle cell anemia. The children's asthma team screens children with major secondary chronic illnesses. If it is determined that they can be safely accommodated at camp, a written release is requested from the physician providing the child's specialty care.

APPLICATION OF TEACHING AND LEARNING PRINCIPLES

Assessment

Sound educational programs are based on assessing learner needs. Parents of campers complete a four-page history prior to camp. In the history, parents are asked to identify the aspect of asthma management they most want the child to master. Parents also identify characteristics of the child that may impact learning, such as difficulty with hearing or vision or attention deficit disorder. In the latter case, parents are instructed to ensure that the child continue medication each day of camp because camp is a structured learning activity.

Two weeks prior to camp, parents and children attend a required orientation. Peak flow and metered-dose inhaler or dry powder inhaler techniques are assessed with each child. Children also complete baseline asthma knowledge and self-efficacy (confidence managing asthma) questionnaires.

The camper's medical history is reviewed with parents. Interactions with the campers and parents provide further opportunities to assess learning needs. The pediatric asthma team supplements these data, when possible, based on learning needs identified during clinic visits.

Learning is Individualized

Counselors receive copies of medical histories of the children assigned to their care and focus individual instruction on identified learning needs. In addition, each child receives a self-management plan called the "RAD plan." The RAD plan uses exciting colors and visuals that fit the theme chosen for the camp session. The child's individual triggers, early warning signs, and medications are listed on the plan. Plans are kept at hand for easy reference by placing them in the child's camp fanny pack. The child is requested to use the plan for the trigger, early warning sign, and medication sessions. Campers are individually counseled regarding how session content applies to their individual management plan. Teachable moments throughout camp activities also provide opportunities for individualizing instruction.

Counselors are encouraged to talk to parents at the end of each camp day. Consultation with the parents provides counselors with the opportunity to clarify issues the child identifies and to share the child's learning progress. Counselors can also use the time to encourage parents to reinforce specific management concepts unique to that child.

Perception – Small groups

Learners must be able to see and hear instruction. Application of this teaching and learning principle is challenging in a camp setting. Camp RAD is held outdoors on the Gulf Coast, where heat, humidity, wind, and competing audio stimuli must be considered in educational planning. The camp has access to an air-conditioned field house with a mirrored aerobic room, small office spaces, and a gymnasium.

Asthma classes are held indoors to improve control of perceptual factors. Children are taught in small groups of six or eight. Each group is assigned class space in a separate area of the field house. Aerobic benches are used as seating and are arranged to direct attention away from the distracting mirrored walls. Where needed, gym mats are used to create walls to separate groups. Classes are scheduled in the morning when a child's attention is best and when field house members are least likely to be using the facilities.

Link Learning to Past Experiences

Children learn best when learning is linked to familiar experiences in their lives. Whenever possible, new asthma content in the camp curriculum is linked to everyday experiences that children understand. For example, the anatomy of the airway is compared to upside down broccoli. Variability of asthma is likened to the weather. The big blast from the peak flow meter is likened to blowing out the candles on the birthday cake. A warning sign is likened to the railroad signal that a train is approaching.

Campers are also asked to interact by contributing their own examples of everyday asthma experience linkages. Children may contribute by identifying that the lungs look like a bunch of grapes or an upside-down tree. Involvement is motivating to children and helps the educator assess accuracy of understanding of important concepts.

Motivation

Learning must be motivating to the learner. Asthma classes are designed as fun activities. Effort is made to avoid terms that campers may associate with school stress. Words such as "class" and "test" are avoided. Rather, staff use terms such as "meeting," "session," or "feedback." Meetings are short, 20 to 30 minutes, and scheduled prior to swimming, soccer, or other camp activities. Counselors rehearse asthma content and work on maintaining children's interest by incorporating expression and enthusiasm in their presentations. Sessions high-light benefits of learning, such as feeling better, playing sports better, or sleeping through the night. Verbal praise is given frequently, and children receive an asthma education award on the final camp day. Children who master application of asthma content are invited back to camp as junior counselor role models. The junior counselor program is highly motivating to the campers and provides a strong incentive to become good asthma managers.

Learning is Interactive

Children do not learn in linear, hierarchical steps. Children's learning is a dynamic, interactive process that flows back and forth as the child matures through developmental stages (Vygotsky, 1989). Effective children's education programs are highly interactive.

Camp counselors provide didactic content in 2-minute segments to allow for interactive opportunities for children. To illustrate, airway anatomy is verbally described while Radical Randy's™ airway is shown as a visual. Children are then encouraged to feel the airway and to feel their own trachea. Younger children trace the body of a camper on paper and then apply parts of the airway in the correct anatomical positions. The function of a miniature bronchiole is described. Children are encouraged to feel the air that flows freely through the open airway. The "meeting" proceeds in an interactive format. Remaining "meetings" are similarly structured. Even concepts such as catching a cold are made interactive through the use of a glitter handshake.

Probably one of the most powerful interactive learning opportunities is the "teachable moment." Teachable moments occur spontaneously at any time in the program. Counselors must remain on alert to capitalize on these opportunities. One such spontaneous moment was a runaway cage ball. A cage ball is a light, 72-inch ball used in camp activities. A gust of wind picked up the ball, blew it out of the campgrounds and down the street toward a ferry depot. In their excitement, campers spontaneously darted after the ball. Some campers experienced exercised-induced asthma symptoms. This was an ideal teaching opportunity because it allowed the educators to directly apply preventive strategies to a real life situation at the moment it was most relevant to the child.

Repetition

Children need repetition of new concepts. The Camp RAD program integrates this learning principle in several ways. Important asthma management concepts are highlighted after each teaching session. The education sessions close with all campers practicing a jingle called the "RAD Rap." Each of seven verses of the RAD Rap highlights the main message of the asthma teaching session. To assure that campers have their verses on hand, the RAD Rap is permanently printed on the backs of their camp T-shirts.

Medication administration and peak flow skills are practiced continually throughout the camp program. Three peak flow meter readings are scheduled into the camp program to provide reinforcement of learning. One-to-two adult-to-camper ratios at these check points provides for intense individual skill reinforcement.

The curriculum is designed around repetition of concepts. The weather metaphor, used to describe the chronic nature of asthma, is repeated in peak flow meter instruction. Peak flow is likened to the weather report because it indicates approaching of stormy asthma before symptoms are experienced. Early warning signs are compared to signs of approaching stormy weather.

The camp skit, (described below), provides more opportunities for repetition of asthma concepts because the children rehearse an asthma-related story throughout the week. The theme of the skit is an asthma management topic such as importance of controller medication or trigger avoidance. Children rehearse the skit each day and present the

play for their parents on the last day of camp. Acting out the role of a cat, dust, or smoke trigger or the role of a peak flow meter or medication provides a dynamic opportunity to reinforce asthma management content through repetition.

LEARNING THROUGH SPORTS

Participation in all activities, including sports, is a key goal of the NAEPP. It is well known that many people with asthma limit physical activity. The camp staff gained more appreciation of the extent of self-imposed activity limitation through their direct work with campers in a natural environment.

Camp RAD is geographically situated on an island that is approximately 3 to 4 miles wide. Children attending the program live on the island or nearby on the mainland. Each year it is astounding to meet school-age children who have lived their lives by the coast but never visited the beach because of the misperception that people with asthma cannot go to the beach.

Other children are frightened by exercised-induced symptoms and therefore avoid sports; still others love sports but perform poorly because they lack instruction in preventive strategies. Some campers report participation limitations imposed by school coaches who do not understand asthma.

Full participation in all activities is a prerequisite for camp attendance. This expectation is clearly communicated to parents and campers prior to camp. Most parents respond that this is one of their personal goals and they are comforted by the knowledge that campers participate in sports under the guidance of a pediatric asthma team. The camp's physician is also a soccer coach and masterfully combines exercise-induced asthma prevention strategies with soccer instruction. Lay coaches are recruited for directing other activities such as martial arts. Participation in the camp program positively impacts their understanding of the activity needs of children with asthma. Coaches come away with an understanding that participation in sports is safe for children with asthma when a few simple guidelines are followed.

Parents report that as a result of guided sports participation and excursions to the beach, many children expand their world and become more physically active after camp by joining sports teams for the first time or improving physical endurance. In fact, two campers achieved outstanding sports recognition. After learning proper use of medication and the values of a slow warm up, one child was admitted to the junior Olympic track and field team. Her brother achieved state ranking in track and field.

Having health professionals swimming, playing soccer, or performing martial arts alongside children with asthma in a natural setting sends a powerful message about the value of sports participation that cannot be delivered in a classroom or clinic setting.

CREATIVE STRATEGIES

Activities

Creative strategies incorporated in the camp education sessions, such as use of metaphors, the three-dimensional anatomical model, and the RAD Rap, are described above. This section describes how creativity is used in camp activities to reinforce asthma education.

Arts and crafts are natural activities to include in a camp program. One arts and crafts period uses art to encourage children to express their feelings about living with asthma. Examples of art projects to enhance expression of feelings include creating self-portraits that portray the camper with and without breathing difficulty, constructing asthma wish boxes, and creating a feeling fish made of individual scales that express the feelings of each camper. A child life specialist experienced in the use of therapeutic play with children with chronic illness guides discussion.

Activities are sometimes created to include asthma management concepts. A favorite with the campers is the treasure hunt. Children living on the Gulf Coast are familiar with stories of the pirate Jean Lafitte and buried treasure. However, most children do not know that Jean Lafitte had a first mate called Atticus who suffered from asthma. On a particularly important pirate raid, Atticus inhaled dust from gunpowder and experienced status asthmaticus. There were no asthma inhalers in those days, so Jean Lafitte was forced to abandon the raid and head for the island where a natural root could be used to help Atticus breathe. The pirates found the root but were repelled by its foul odor. Jean Lafitte recognized that the odor was a perfect barrier to keep others away from his treasure, so he buried his loot at this site. A staff member, dressed as Atticus, enhances the treasure hunt. Atticus accompanies the children on their adventure. Children respond to clues to help Atticus breathe easier and each response leads them closer to the treasure. The treasure hunt can be adapted in many ways. A camp session with a space theme incorporated an alien landing into the treasure hunt.

The "Information Super Highway" was created for the computer themed camp session. A winding jogging track made an ideal site to place small mats that represented life-sized spaces of a board game. Information required to advance along the board game were correct responses to an asthma puzzler. In addition to advancing on the highway, correct responses were rewarded with the opportunity to "dunk the doctor" in a water box. Needless to say, dunking the doctor was motivating!

Obstacle courses are a common camp activity. A creative twist to enhance reinforcement of airway anatomy was added to the obstacle race by constructing a life-sized airway from tunnels. Small 1½ ft (0.46m) and large 2½ ft (0.76m) play tunnels were purchased from a recreational store. The large tunnel, or main airway, was situated 20 ft (6.1m) from the start/finish line. The small tunnel (bronchiole) was placed 10 ft (3.05m) from the main airway. Hula-hoops were used to frame netting that represented air sacs. They were situated 10 ft from the bronchioles. Black balls (carbon dioxide) filled the air sacs. Children separated into two teams—one at the right and one at the left airway. They were given a white ball (oxygen) at the start line. The goal was to race to the air sac and replace the carbon dioxide with oxygen.

The Skit

Activities for the children are fun and solidify their understanding of asthma, but parents are missing from this educational experience. In fact, some parents interpret the term "self-management" as meaning that children should independently manage their asthma. These parents disengage from care. Use of the term "self-management" is actively discouraged at camp and staff use "partnership" in its place.

The asthma team uses an innovative approach to foster parent involvement. The skit was designed to engage parents in asthma education in a fun manner. The team's value, that parents are partners in care, is central to the camp skit. At camp enrollment, parents are informed that the children will be performing for them and receiving awards on the last day of camp. Their attendance is expected. Importance of being present for the children, rather than asthma education, is the message that is given to the parents.

Skits are written to highlight one or two aspects of asthma management in a way that has appeal to children. A skit with an alien landing in a silver space ship provides an exciting event for the campers. This skit is enhanced by a life-sized silver space ship with flashing lights and costuming for the alien. The alien, a break-dancer, is friendly and shows the children how dancing is done on Jupiter and Mars. As the alien performs he starts wheezing and coughing because of the pollution in the Earth's atmosphere. The campers recognize the symptoms as asthma and teach the alien how to manage his breathing so that he can return home to Jupiter. This skit highlights recognition of early warning signs.

The skit, "Mr. Ree and the Trigger Detectives," is written with a focus on trigger avoidance strategies. Mr. Ree, a much loved drama teacher and friend of the mayor, becomes ill after purchasing a new home. He suspects that he is experiencing asthma, so he calls upon his students who are graduates of Camp RAD. In typical dramatic fashion, Mr. Ree sends a cryptic message to the camper's private clubhouse. Mr. Ree has an odd quirk—he is very frugal. He needs help immediately so he arranges for transportation for the campers. He sends his limosine, which is split down the middle to save gas!

The campers are stirred by the cryptic contents of the message and anticipate a mystery. They gather their detective equipment and board the limosine. Upon arrival at Mr. Ree's house they are upset to see that he is very sick. The campers rise to the occasion and become trigger detectives. They explain to Mr. Ree that new houses do not breathe well and are trigger treasures. After identifying and removing the offending substances, Mr. Ree breathes easier. News of his recovery reaches the Mayor who presents the campers with an award. A real former city mayor, who actively supports asthma programs in the community, plays the role of mayor.

The importance of taking daily controller medication is the main message of the skit, "Rapturous Randy and the Beast." This skit is inspired by the fairy tale, *Beauty and the Beast.* In typical fairy tale fashion, Rapturous Randy's family loses all of their wealth and are banished to a hovel in the forest to eke out a living. The mean sisters leave Rapturous Randy in the forest searching for nuts and mushrooms to make mushroom mush for dinner. Rapturous Randy becomes weary and lies down beneath a mossy tree to nap. The trees are animated and talk about their pride that Rapturous Randy has chosen them to protect her. They soon become concerned because they hear a whistling sound in her breathing. The forest fairy, who has magical fairy powder, is summoned.

When the fairy arrives she explains that the moss and dirt have caused Rapturous Randy to develop the whistling breathing. She breaks off a branch from the mossy old tree, blows through it to create a hollow spacer and blows fairy powder into Rapturous Randy. Rapturous Randy awakens and the fairy gives her preventive powder with the instructions to take it every day. She further explains that there once was a Prince Charming who developed the whistling breathing but he refused to take the daily fairy powder. As his breathing became more difficult, he turned blue and his face became pinched from the work of breathing. Eventually, he became a Beast. The fairy told Rapturous Randy that she still had her beauty and could retain her beauty if she took her daily medicine. Rapturous Randy promises to take her daily controller medicine.

The tale goes on with Rapturous Randy eventually meeting the Beast. She is successful in convincing him to take the breathing medicine. He is transformed back into Prince Charming and they live happily ever after.

Parental attendance at skits is high. Parents enjoy the humor of the stories and they love watching the children perform, but they also learn important asthma concepts. Feedback from parents include statements indicating that they did not realize how much there was to learn about asthma, or that they need to obtain more information because their children understand asthma better than they do.

IMPACT ON COMMUNITY RELATIONSHIPS AND INTERDISCIPLINARY TEAMWORK

The camp program uses a variety of resources. Many of these resources are obtained through in-kind donations. Relationships have strengthened with the community as businesses, professionals, and media personnel partner to support the camp. Area restaurants provide lunches for the campers and staff. Photography, T-shirt, and activity specialists; theater personnel; and reporters all contribute needed services. Asthma is so prevalent that many of the business managers and professionals have close friends or family members who have asthma, so they are eager to support the program.

Health profession students serving as counselors find that the camp as a clinical experience provides them with a rare opportunity to work as peers within an interdisciplinary team. Living with team members in the field while providing direct care to children who are learning to control a chronic illness is a powerful experience in teamwork. Relationships continue long after camp is over.

EVALUATION OF CAMP PROGRAMS

Evaluation is a core value of the camp program. Evaluation identifies strengths of the program as well as areas that need modification. Measurement of outcomes provides objective data on the impact of the program. This information is important to program planners, administrators who provide organizational support, and funding agencies.

Despite the current emphasis on evidence-based data in planning healthcare programs, six reviews of the literature failed to produce any reports of randomized controlled trials of the impact of camp programs on asthma outcomes for children. Lack of controlled studies may be due to the fact that it is very difficult to design blinded studies of camp programs. Randomized controlled studies would make an important contribution to our understanding of the effect of camp programs. Asthma symptoms tend to improve as children grow, and thus the effect of uncontrolled studies of asthma camps must consider the possibility that some improvement in outcomes is related to influence of growth on asthma. Nevertheless, the day camp described in this chapter is outcome-based. Data collected are significant, showing stable results over an 11-year period. Long-term stability of findings indicates sound programming.

Campers have consistently shown significant asthma knowledge and self-efficacy gains after camp and effects continue to be demonstrated 6 months after the program (Meng, Tiernan, Bernier, & Brooks, 1998). Twelve months after camp, data are collected on frequency of missed school days, hospitalizations, emergency room (ER) and urgent care visits, and the parents' perception of child asthma management and activity tolerance. Statistically significant differences are documented each year. The impact was dramatic the first year but was diluted thereafter due to a high rate of returning campers.

In addition to formal evaluation campers, parents, students, staff, and university personnel provide informal feedback on the value of the camp program. Camp RAD has generated a high degree of satisfaction among the various groups that it influences.

THE NURSE'S ROLE IN SUPPORTING CHILDREN ATTENDING CAMP

Nurses can support asthma camps in several ways. Nurses can refer campers, educate families about the benefits of camp programs, and participate directly by volunteering at camp. High-risk children (children who visit the ER, are hospital-ized, make urgent care visits, or frequently miss school due to asthma) should be referred to camps. High-risk children are likely to lack continuity of care and may not receive adequate asthma education during urgent care visits. Many of the families of these children have no understanding of asthma camps unless a nurse or healthcare worker who provides direct care advocates for them. Families may be reluctant to pursue enrolling the child because of financial reasons. The nurse should obtain information about camp registration fees. Pharmaceutical companies or other donors commonly provide camping scholarships for children in need.

Some families are unclear about the nature of asthma camps. The nurse can provide accurate information regarding benefits of these programs. Children learn to apply asthma management concepts at camp. This learning is seen in reduced ER visits, urgent care visits, and missed school days. Feedback from parents also indicates that children are more responsible in taking medications and peak flow measurements after the camp experience. Some parents report that children have greater activity tolerance or acquire new skills such as acting. A number of children selected healthcare professions as a career choice after attending camp.

Nurses may wish to participate directly in a camp program as a way of supporting children and their families or as a way of advancing their own understanding of asthma. In these cases, contact should be made directly with local camp directors.

SUMMARY

Camps for children with asthma provide a unique opportunity to provide asthma education in an applied, developmentally appropriate fashion. Effective camp programs have a clear mission statement, are theory-based, incorporate consensus guidelines and principles of learning, and utilize professionally prepared staff. School-age children with moderate persistent asthma who lack knowledge of asthma management are most likely to benefit from a camp program. Learning in a camp setting is effective because knowledge is applied in a concrete fashion using actual experiences. Creative strategies that enhance learning are easily integrated into a camp program. Camp programs have the potential to indirectly increase parent asthma knowledge and increase parent, child, staff, and community satisfaction with care.

CASE STUDY

Mrs. Smith is a single parent with two children who have asthma. Ted, age 9, and Sara, age 7, have moderate persistent asthma and are managed with fluticasone on a daily basis and albuterol as needed. They regularly attend the community clinic but are seen by a different physician at each visit. Mrs. Smith is pleased with their care because since starting the controller medication the children have experienced a decrease in the number of days of missed school. In the past they missed approximately 30 days of school, but now they miss only 15 days per year.

Recently, the school nurse informed Mrs. Smith that Ted and Sara make frequent visits to the school clinic for rescue medication and that 15 school absences is excessive. The school nurse provides Mrs. Smith with a brochure and contact information about a local asthma camp. The nurse discusses the educational program at the camp and its impact on improved asthma control. Mrs. Smith notes that the camp fees are outside the limits of her budget. The school nurse places a call to the camp and learns that scholarships are available. She puts Mrs. Smith in touch with another parent who has children that attended the camp.

Ted and Sara attend camp and have a great time. Mrs. Smith attends the skit and is delighted to see Ted and Sara performing as the cat and dust triggers.

One year after camp, Mrs. Smith is contacted as part of the outcome evaluation plan. Mrs. Smith is delighted with the effects of the program. Ted and Sara have missed no school, have had no urgent care visits, sleep through the night for the first time in years, and hardly ever use their rescue medication "as if they don't have asthma any more!" Mrs. Smith is asked what specifically made the difference. She responds that the children came home every night with exciting stories about all the wonderful things they were learning about their bodies. They started measuring peak flow and taking controller medication more regularly. The children also identified triggers in the home and asked Mrs. Smith to get rid of the cat and carpet. Mrs. Smith notes that she never learned these things at the clinic, but she complied with the children's requests. She was particularly horrified when the carpet removal revealed hidden dust and dirt. The problem was so extensive that the children had to move in with a relative until the new tile was installed. Mrs. Smith credits camp with a dramatic change in her families' life. Prior to camp she had no concept of comprehensive asthma care or the potential for improved control.

Answer the following study questions, writing your responses on a separate sheet of paper. Compare your responses with the answers located at the end of the chapter.

1. What characteristics made Ted and Sara priority candidates for asthma camp?

2. What was the primary factor that motivated Mrs. Smith to enroll her children in camp?

3. What principle of learning probably had the greatest impact on Ted and Sara's learning?

4. How does Mrs. Smith's response to Ted and Sara's pre-camp asthma control compare to asthma management goals?

5. In addition to school, what are other settings in which the nurse can advocate for children to attend camp?

Answers to Case Study

1. Several characteristics made Ted and Sara priority candidates for camp: history of moderate persistent asthma, excessive school absences, overuse of albuterol, and their ages.

2. Advocacy of the school nurse was the key factor in enrolling the children in camp. Especially critical was the support the nurse gave Mrs. Smith in obtaining scholarship information and speaking to another parent familiar with the program.

3. Interactive learning is the educational principle that probably has the greatest impact on the children's learning. As it happened, the children were assigned roles in the skit that matched their triggers and they actively played out the affects of these triggers.

4. Mrs. Smith noted partial progress in asthma control with inconsistent use of medication before camp. Her expectations were low, so she was satisfied with care. Her response is typical of many individuals with asthma. Expectations consistently need to be set higher.

5. Nurses in other settings provide care for high-risk children with asthma. Children admitted to the hospital or visiting the ER or urgent care clinics should be considered for referral to camp programs.

EXAM QUESTIONS

CHAPTER 15
Questions 93-97

93. Principles of learning that enhance asthma education are

    a. link curriculum to everyday experiences the learner can relate to.

    b. using only visual content in the instruction.

    c. providing predominantly verbal content in the instruction.

    d. assuring that content is not repetitious.

94. Teaching the child with asthma to participate in sports is best accomplished by

    a. classroom instruction.

    b. physician encouragement in the clinic setting.

    c. demonstrating improved pulmonary function after training.

    d. doing a slow warm-up and playing soccer with the child.

95. Creative learning strategies described in this chapter best illustrate the teaching and learning principle of

    a. interactive learning.

    b. ability to see and hear instruction.

    c. assessment of the learner.

    d. hierarchial learning.

96. Asthma education in a camp setting is *best* accomplished through

    a. systematic group instruction.

    b. opportunities to provide individual instruction.

    c. encouraging parents to reinforce learning at home.

    d. a combination of group and individual instruction.

97. Children and families are most likely to learn about benefits of asthma camp programs through

    a. newspaper notices.

    b. explanations from a nurse.

    c. physician referral.

    d. information obtained independently.

REFERENCES

Erikson, E. (1963). *Childhood and society.* (2nd ed.) New York: W. W. Norton.

Meng, A., Tiernan, K., Bernier, M. J., & Brooks, E. G. (1998). An evaluation of the effectiveness of an asthma day camp. *The American Journal of Maternal Child Nursing, 23*, 300-306.

National Asthma Education and Prevention Program. (1997). Expert panel report 2. *Guidelines for the diagnosis and management of asthma.* (NIH Publication No. 97-4051). Bethesda, MD: National Institutes of Health, National Heart, Lung, and Blood Institute. Available online at www.nhlbi.nih.gov/guidelines/asthma/index.pdf

National Asthma Education and Prevention Program. (2003). Expert Panel Report: *Guidelines for the diagnosis and management of asthma: Update on selected topics 2002.* (NIH Publication No. 02-5074). Bethesda, MD: National Institutes of Health, National Heart, Lung and Blood Institute. Available online at http://www.nhlbi.nih.gov/guidelines/asthma/index.html

Piaget, J. (1969). *Theory of Stages in Cognitive Development.* New York: McGraw-Hill.

Vygotsky, L. (1989). Concrete human psychology. *Social Psychology, 27*, 53-77.

CHAPTER 16

RELAXATION AND ALTERNATIVE THERAPIES IN THE TREATMENT OF ASTHMA

CHAPTER OBJECTIVE

Upon completion of this chapter, the reader will be able to identify the nurse's role in educating patients with asthma and their families about alternative therapies and their impact on asthma.

LEARNING OBJECTIVES

After studying this chapter, the reader will be able to

1. recognize the prevalence of using alternative therapies to treat asthma.

2. identify alternative therapies most commonly used by patients with asthma.

3. recognize potential benefits and risks associated with alternative therapies.

4. state the cost of alternative therapy to the patient.

5. provide scientifically sound education about alternative therapies to patients and families.

OVERVIEW

Although not a mainstay of therapy, use of alternative therapies by patients with asthma warrants discussion because of its increasing popularity. Use of alternative therapies is so prevalent that nurses can expect to provide care to a large number of patients who use therapies other than tradi-

tional medicine. These therapies may impact the delivery of medical care, so it is important to ask about history of use of alternative therapies in the nursing assessment. The nurse has a responsibility to those patients who use other therapies to provide them with accurate information about the safety and potential adverse interactions with traditional medical care. This chapter focuses specifically on the use of alternative therapies in the treatment of asthma.

PREVALENCE OF USE OF ALTERNATIVE THERAPIES

Alternative therapy is a poorly defined term. It includes a wide assortment of treatments such as herbal remedies, homeopathic products, chiropractic and massage treatments, relaxation techniques and yoga, to name a few. Between 1990 and 1997 it is estimated that there was a five-fold increase in the use of herbal treatments among adults in the United States. Healthcare providers typically underestimate use of alternative therapies (Lanski, Greenwald, Perkins, & Simon, 2003).

A telephone survey of adults with asthma and rhinosinusitis indicated that use of alternative therapies is much more prevalent than previously thought and that use among this population is increasing (Blanc, Trupin, Earnest, Katz, Yelin, & Eisner, 2001). Almost half (42%) of 127 adults reported using alternative therapies specifically to treat breathing or nasal symptoms in the past year. Especially disturbing is the report that half of those using alternative therapy had no prescription medications.

Alternative therapies are increasing in popularity because they are perceived as natural remedies and therefore are viewed as safe. Some patients use these therapies to avoid visits to the physician or to avoid use of steroid medication, which they may view as unsafe. Friends and family members, rather than scientific sources, are primary providers of information about alternative therapies. The most commonly used alternative therapy is herbal remedies. These remedies are thought by many to be benign. Because herbs are considered a dietary product, their regulation is under the control of the Dietary Supplement Health and Education Act of 1994. This act requires appropriate labeling only. Consumer information on safety of herbals is lacking because the Act does not require demonstration of safety or efficacy before the product is placed on the market. Only after the product is on the market and adverse events are reported does the herbal product come under safety regulation of the Food and Drug Administration (FDA) (Lanski et al., 2003).

The most commonly used herbal remedy among adults with asthma is ephedra. Adults with asthma also commonly use caffeinated beverages to treat breathing or nasal symptoms (Blanc et al., 2001). Caffeine is pharmacologically related to the methylxanthines (theophylline) and does have some bronchodilator properties. Before the advent of modern medicines, caffeinated beverages were commonly used to treat asthma.

Patients tend to use more than one alternative therapy. Homeopathy, massage, aromatherapy, and acupuncture are commonly reported. Decision to use alternative therapy is not related to the patient's severity of symptoms, but women (Blanc et al., 2001) and those with at least some college education are more likely to report using alternative therapy (Lanski et al. 2003).

In interviews performed in a pediatric emergency room, less than half of parents who gave their children herbal remedies said they reported using the herbal therapies to their pysicians. Reasons for failing to disclose this information included forgetting or thinking it was unimportant. Several parents who did try to share this information were told the physician had no knowledge of the product or were told they were abusing their child. These responses discourage reporting and are potentially dangerous because information about the patient's history is incomplete.

COMMONLY USED ALTERNATIVE THERAPIES FOR ASTHMA

Parents who gave their children herbal products tended to use three or more herbal products. The most common were aloe plant or juice, echinacea, and sweet oil. The most dangerous combination was ephedra and albuterol. Unusual products included turpentine (for worms), pine needles, and cowchips. Other less commonly used products included ginko, ginseng, goldenseal, and valerian root. The most common reasons for administering herbals were upper respiratory infection, cuts, relaxation, or to stimulate the immune response (Lanski et al., 2003). The latter reason is particularly interesting because the cause of asthma can be thought of as overstimulation of the immune system, particularly the Th2 helper cells. Nevertheless, parents interviewed thought the herbals had no side effects or drug interactions.

Other commonly used alternative therapies include acupuncture, homeopathy, ayurvedic medicine, osteopathy and chiropractic manipulations, hypnosis, biofeedback, (National Heart, Lung, and Blood Institute [NHLBI]/World Health Organization [WHO], 2003), fasting, dietary supplements, aromatherapy, hopi candles, and relaxation (Bosquet, van Cauwenberge, & Khaltaev, 2001).

Acupuncture

Acupuncture has been used to treat asthma. There are some reports on its benefit, but these reports are from uncontrolled trials. There is no scientific evidence that acupuncture improves asthma outcomes. Acupuncture is difficult to study because of difficulties blinding control groups to the intervention. Most of the data on acupuncture are imbedded in centuries of experience as described in the Chinese literature, but this body of literature is difficult to examine. Recently, four randomized controlled studies and three placebo-controlled studies evaluated the effect of acupuncture on asthma but found no effect. Serious side effects, however, have been documented and include pneumothorax, hepatitis and other infections, death, burns, and endocarditis. At least one death was attributed to a fatal asthma attack while the patient was under the needles (Györik & Brutsche, 2004).

Traditional Chinese medicine claims asthma benefits from acupuncture. Acupuncture does have some effect on inflammatory cells but results are not lasting. Critics point out that Western studies concluding no benefit from this modality have omitted a personalization component of acupuncture. One study that implemented personalized placement of acupuncture needles according to the patient's symptoms found no long-term benefit. There are some data that acupuncture improves symptoms during an acute attack, but the reduction in airway resistance is short term and less than what is achieved with rescue medication. Despite claims, no long-term benefit has been documented (Shapira et al., 2001).

Traditional Chinese medicine uses acupuncture holistically in combination with diet, herbs, and lifestyle changes. Acupuncture is rarely used this way in the West, and the holistic approach is very difficult to study. The official position of the con-

sensus group is that acupuncture is not indicated for the treatment of asthma (NHLBI/WHO, 2003).

Herbal Therapies

Plants have been used for illness since the beginning of time. Herbal preparations are known to have pharmacologic effects. For this reason, many modern medications are derived from plants. Several drugs, including commonly used asthma medications, have roots in herbal remedies. Examples of asthma medications with herbal roots include cromones (cromoyln sodium), beta-agonists, anticholinergics, and methylxanthines (theophylline) (NHLBI/WHO, 2003).

There is some evidence that herbals may have an effect on asthma. Dried ivy showed some effect on decreasing airway resistance, but only one of three trials included a control group. A randomized controlled study conducted in China combined a decoction of xiaoqinglong with fluticasone. Statistically greater improvement in lung function was found with the herbal-drug combination than with fluticasone alone. Another well-controlled study found that the herbal complex, saiboku, improved airway hyperresponsiveness and asthma symptoms after four weeks of treatment three times per day. A recent study conducted jointly by John Hopkins University, Mount Sinai School of Medicine, and the Peking Union Medical College found that a Chinese herbal preparation (MSSM-002) suppressed airway hyperreactivity and inflammation without suppressing Th1, the cell involved in the protective immune response. This herbal preparation may have a potential benefit in asthma (Li et al., 2004).

Well-designed, controlled studies demonstrating benefit from herbal therapy are few and insufficient in number to recommend use of herbs to treat asthma. Despite the public belief that herbals are safe because they are natural products, the pharmacological activity of herbs makes them potentially dangerous. For example, the herb, comfrey, is sold as a tea or root powder but contains toxins and have been associated with veno-occlusive disease (NHLBI/WHO, 2003). The combination of ephedra and albuterol is dangerous (Lanski et al., 2003). Ephedra, also called ma huang, is commonly contained in dietary supplements as a weight loss, energy enhancing, or sports enhancing product. Ephedra is a naturally occurring plant substance. Its active ingredient is ephedrine. Ephedrine when chemically synthesized is regulated as a drug. Ephedra has many side effects and drug interactions. It has been linked to at least 100 deaths. Ephedra raises blood pressure, stresses the cardiovascular system, and is linked to stroke and myocardial infarction. The FDA issued a consumer alert on the safety of ephedra in 2003 (U.S. Food and Drug Administration, 2003).

Herbal remedies have the potential to cause contact dermatitis because of their sensitizing properties. Various preparations have caused organ toxicity involving the liver, kidneys, and heart. Some herbals products may even have carcinogenic properties (Niggemann & Gruber, 2003).

Use of herbals in adults with asthma has been associated with increased risk of hospitalization. It is not clear if hospitalization is a direct result of herbal use or if use of herbals is related to lack of use of anti-inflammatory medication (Györik & Brutsche, 2004). There are at least 24 cases of interstitial pneumonitis related to herbal therapy (Györik & Brutsche, 2004).

Because of their popularity, many people are seeking information on herbals. The World Wide Web provides a rich source of information advocating use of herbal therapy, but unfortunately, most of the Web-based information advocating use of herbs is uncontrolled.

Homeopathy

Homeopathy began in Germany over 200 years ago and is widely practiced in many countries. Homeopathic practitioners describe homeopathy as a natural, scientific form of medicine that treats the mind and body. Minute amounts of medicines, commonly herbals, are used with the promise of long lasting results or cures. Homeopathic preparations for treatment of asthma that is triggered by dust mite and grass pollen have been tested, but study methodology was poor and no conclusions were drawn (Bousquet et al., 2001). A couple of recent well designed studies found no benefit but also no risks (Györik & Brutsche, 2004). Homeopathy is not recommended for the treatment of asthma (NHLBI/WHO, 2003).

Ayurvedic Medicine

Ayurvedic is a Sanskrit word that means, "knowledge of life." Ayurvedic medicine has been practiced in India for thousands of years. It has 20 separate components that include transcendental meditation, herbals, pulse diagnosis, and yoga. It has been used to treat asthma but there are no data to support its use (Bousquet et al., 2001).

Breathing Exercises and Yoga

Breathing exercises and yoga offer the strongest hope for effective alternative therapies in the treatment of asthma. Buteyko is a breath holding technique practiced in Russia, the United Kingdom, Australia, and New Zealand. One study reported improvement in asthma symptoms with buteyko, but the study was poorly designed and discouraged subjects from using rescue medication (Györik & Brutsche, 2004). On the other hand, breathing retraining may have some impact on asthma. Patients with asthma sometimes have functional breathing problems that result in breathlessness, chest pain, anxiety, and fatigue. These patients overbreathe or hyperventilate, so the dysfunctional breathing is referred to as "hyperventilation syndrome." Clinical findings include irregular breathing, sighing, and use of the upper chest rather than the diaphragm for breathing. Patients with asthma and dysfunctional breathing who were taught diaphragmatic breathing and practiced it daily reported improvement in quality of life but no change in anxiety (Thomas et al., 2003). Two randomized controlled trials of inspiratory muscle training resulted in decreased dyspnea and decreased use of bronchodilators after 20 weeks of training but small sample size and possible selection bias limit ability to generalize the findings (Györik & Brutsche, 2004).

Sahaja yoga is a traditional system of meditation based on yoga principles. A randomly controlled trial showed limited benefit on asthma symptoms and airway hyperresponsiveness after 4 months of treatment, but the effect was short term (Manocha, Marks, Kenchington, Peters, & Salome, 2002). One type of yoga breathing exercise, pranayama, may have a small affect on histamine reactivity but it does not have an affect on other asthma parameters (NHLBI/WHO, 2003).

Diet

Current research is addressing the question of dietary influence on the increasing prevalence of asthma. If this is the case, modification of diet may have the potential to reduce disease prevalence and severity. An epidemiological study showed a correlation between asthma mortality in males and increased sales of table salt. Several studies showed a small but significant improvement in asthma symptoms in men, but not women, on a low-sodium diet (T'Veen, Sterk, & Bel, 2000).

Selenium, a trace element with nutritional properties, may have a slight, nonsignificant effect on asthma but cannot be recommended (T'Veen, Sterk, & Bel, 2000). Epidemiological studies suggest an association between fish oil and asthma symptoms but controlled studies do not support the association (T'Veen, Sterk & Bel, 2000; Györik & Brutsche, 2004). Serum magnesium levels are known to be low in patients with asthma and may be further lowered by use of beta-agonists. Data on the benefit of magnesium replacement conflict.

Effect of vitamins on asthma has been explored to a limited extent. Data do not support use of vitamin B_{12}. There are conflicting data on vitamin B_6 but the largest study to date showed no effect. Vitamin C supplementation is not considered effective but at the most may have a slight effect on exercise-induced asthma (T'Veen, Sterk, & Bel, 2000). Antioxidants may have a role in asthma therapy, but there is currently insufficient evidence to support their use (Györik & Brutsche, 2004).

Relaxation

Relaxation therapy for patients with asthma is based on the observation that a person with asthma has a different airway response to stress than a person without asthma. In a healthy person, stress reduces airway resistance. The opposite effect occurs in a person with asthma. Likewise, exercise causes bronchodilation in a healthy person but causes airway narrowing in a person with asthma. Difficulty breathing causes anxiety. It is thought that relaxation can help reduce the stress associated with acute asthma symptoms. Some data report that progressive muscle relaxation improves lung function in patients with asthma, but it is generally considered that relaxation alone does not produce clinically significant improvement in asthma. However, relaxation is useful when it is combined with a comprehensive self-management plan (Huntley, White, & Ernst, 2002). Relaxation has the disadvantage that it has to be practiced frequently.

Anecdotal data from use of relaxation in a camp setting indicate that some children, but not others, are receptive to relaxation therapy. Children who were receptive reported anxiety or were noted by parents or the health team to be anxious. Although specific outcomes of this therapy were not measured, children selected for relaxation reported feeling calmer. Anecdotal reports from parents indicated that a few children continued to practice relaxation at home on a daily basis and perceived that it was beneficial. It may be that relaxation therapy is selectively therapeutic for patients with asthma.

Writing

Adults with asthma were asked to spend 20 minutes, three times per week writing about stressful life events. A comparison control group wrote about emotionally neutral events. Two weeks after beginning the writing, improvements in pulmonary function were noted in the group that wrote about stressful events. These changes persisted at 4 months. The reason for the improvement was not understood, but it was suggested that writing might alter cognition and memory of stressful events in a manner that facilitates coping (Smyth, Stone, Hurewitz, & Kaell, 1999). This is an interesting finding, particularly when one considers that the writing intervention is in the opposite direction of the goals of relaxation therapy. Perhaps strategies need to be tailored to different subpopulations of patients with asthma.

Other Alternative Therapies

Despite claims of benefit, there is no evidence that osteopathy or chiropractic medicine benefits patients with asthma. Reports on the use of hypnosis, behavioral modification, and biofeedback are scarce and contradictory (NHLBI/WHO, 2003). Manual treatments include massage, chest percussion, shaking, and vibration. Five randomized controlled trials showed no evidence of benefit from these therapies. Positive and negative air ionizers have been widely advertised but have shown no benefit in asthma (Györik & Brutsche, 2004).

COST OF ALTERNATIVE THERAPIES

It is estimated that adults in the United States spend $27 billion on alternative therapies annually (Györik & Brutsche, 2004). This represents out-of-pocket costs because insurance generally does not cover the cost of alternative therapy. This figure also does not represent costs of treatment of side effects related to alternative therapy, or asthma

exacerbations due to lack of use of controller medication when using herbal therapies.

Patients' search for alternative therapies may represent lack of satisfaction with traditional medicine and frustration with chronicity of asthma symptoms. Given popularity and high cost, it is acknowledged in the medical community that well designed clinical trials are needed to evaluate effect of alternative therapies.

THE NURSE'S ROLE IN EDUCATING THE PATIENT

The nurse should ask patients and families about the use of alternative therapies as a routine part of the nursing assessment. Failure to ask the question results in inadequate information and missed educational opportunities. The nurse should create a climate of trust to encourage sharing of information.

It is impossible to be informed about all alternative therapies, but the nurse should be aware of commonly used therapies, especially those used by the population served in the nurse's practice. Most patients appreciate an honest response if the practitioner is not familiar with a particular therapy. However, the nurse should follow-up this situation by researching the product and providing the patient with advice.

The nurse has the obligation to provide patients and families with scientifically sound information on the use of alternative therapies. The nurse should monitor updates from the National Asthma Education and Prevention Program or other consensus groups. Therapies that are potentially harmful, such as the use of ephedra, should be discouraged. The safety of inhaled corticosteroids should be reinforced if this is a factor in selecting alternative therapies. Harmless therapies may have a psychotherapeutic effect, but the patient should be informed of their lack of benefit in treating asthma because they may be expensive. Nurses should consider the potential benefit of relaxation therapy for patients who experience anxiety with asthma exacerbations. When referring patients with asthma for relaxation training, communicate the importance of practicing relaxation sitting, rather than lying down to the relaxation therapist. Sitting upright facilitates breathing, especially during an acute attack. Lying down makes breathing more difficult.

SUMMARY

The use of alternative therapies by patients with asthma is becoming increasingly popular, especially among those with college education. Use of alternative therapies is underreported to healthcare providers. Some therapies, especially herbals with bioactive ingredients, may be harmful, but consumer safety information on such products is generally lacking. There are few well-designed studies on alternative therapies. Although some therapies show small potential benefit, there are insufficient data to recommend most therapies. Among alternative approaches, some forms of breathing exercises and relaxation appear to hold the greatest potential for benefit. The nursing role is to assess patient use of alternative therapies and to provide accurate information on such therapies to the patient and family.

EXAM QUESTIONS

CHAPTER 16
Questions 98-100

98. A commonly used herbal remedy that is dangerous for patients with asthma is

    a. ephedra.

    b. cromone.

    c. echinacea.

    d. ginseng.

99. A therapy that has shown improvement in lung function in patients with asthma, when combined with traditional asthma care is

    a. biofeedback.

    b. hypnosis.

    c. relaxation.

    d. acupuncture.

100. On a yearly basis, the amount Americans spend on alternative remedies is

    a. $25 million.

    b. $500 million

    c. $27 billion.

    d. $100 billion.

This concludes the final examination.

REFERENCES

Blanc, P., Trupin, L., Earnest, G., Katz, P., Yelin, E., & Eisner, M. (2001). Alternative therapies among adults with a reported diagnosis of asthma or rhinosinusitis. *Chest, 120*, 1461-1467.

Bosquet, J., van Cauwenberge, P., & Khaltaev, N. (2001). Allergic rhinitis and its impact on asthma (ARIA) in collaboration with the World Health Organization (WHO). *Journal of Allergy and Clinical Immunology, 108*, (Suppl), S147-S336.

Györik, S. & Brutsche, M. (2004). Complementary and alternative medicine for bronchial asthma: Is there new evidence? *Current Opinion in Pulmonary Medicine, 10*, 37-43.

Huntley, A., White, A., & Ernst, E. (2002). Relaxation therapies for asthma: A systematic review. *Thorax, 57*, 127-131.

Lanski, S., Greenwald, M., Perkins, A., & Simon, H. (2003). Herbal therapy use in a pediatric emergency department population: Expect the unexpected. *Pediatrics, 111*, 981-985.

Li, X., Zhang, T., Sampson, H., Zou, Z., Beyer, K., Wen, M., et al. (2004). The potential use of Chinese herbal medicines in treating allergic asthma. *Annals of Allergy, Asthma and Immunology, 93*(2) (Supplement 1), S35-S44.

Manocha, R., Marks, G., Kenchington, P., Peters, D., & Salome, C. (2002). Sahaja yoga in the management of moderate to severe asthma: A randomized controlled trial. *Thorax, 57*, 110-115.

National Heart, Lung, and Blood Institute/World Health Organization. (2003). *Global initiative for asthma: Global strategy for asthma management and prevention.* (NIH Publication No. 02-3659). Retrieved September 12, 2002 from http://www.ginasthma.com

Niggemann, B. & Gruber, C. (2003). Side effects of complementary and alternative medicine. *Allergy, 58*(8), 707-716.

Shapira, M., Berkman, N., Ben-David, G., Avital, A., Bardach, E., & Breuer, R. (2001). Short-term acupuncture therapy is of no benefit in patients with moderate persistent asthma. *Chest, 121*, 1396-1400.

Smyth, J., Stone, A., Hurewitz, A., & Kaell, A. (1999). Effects of writing about stressful experiences on symptom reduction in patients with asthma or rheumatoid arthritis: A randomized trial. *Journal of the American Medical Association, 281*(14), 1304-1309.

Thomas, M., McKinley, R., Freeman, E., Foy, C., Prodger, P., & Price, D. (2003). Breathing retraining for dysfunctional breathing in asthma: A randomized controlled trial. *Thorax, 58*, 110-115.

T'Veen, J., Sterk, P., & Bel, E. (2000). Alternative strategies in the treatment of bronchial asthma. *Clinical and Experimental Allergy, 30*(1), 16-33.

U.S. Food and Drug Administration. (2003). *Consumer alert: FDA plans regulation prohibiting sale of ephedra-containing dietary supplements and advises consumers to stop using these products.* Retrieved January 9, 2005, from http://www.fda.gov/oc/initiatives/ephedra

RESOURCES

ASTHMA RESOURCES ON THE WORLD WIDE WEB

American Academy of Allergy and Immunology
www.aaaai.org

American Lung Association
www.lungusa.org/asthma/
A free stop smoking program is available through this site.

American Thoracic Society – Medical Section of the American Lung Association
www.thoracic.org

Association of Asthma Educators
www.asthmaeducators.org

Asthma and Allergy Foundation of America
www.aafa.org

Asthma and Allergy Network/Mothers of Asthmatics, Inc.
www.aanma.org

Asthma Coalition of Texas
www.texasasthma.org
An asthma resource center for healthcare providers and the public (The reader may wish to locate his or her own state asthma coalition site.)

Asthma Clinical Research Network (ACRN)
www.acrn.org
An excellent resource for readable asthma management plans.

Daily Pollen Count
www.pollen.com
Pollen counts for the entire United States are updated daily.

Global Initiative for Asthma
www.ginasthma.com

Keep Kids Healthy
www.keepkidshealthy.com/asthma/index.html
Allows the user to create a personal color-coded peak flow meter log.

Legacy Products, Inc.
www.legacyproductsinc.com
Provides information on the three-dimensional anatomical asthma teaching doll.

National Asthma Education and Prevention Program - National Heart, Lung, and Blood Institute Information Center
www.nhlbi.nih.gov/guidelines/asthma/asthgdln.htm

Omron Health Care
www.omronhealthcare.com
Provides information on small hand-held nebulizers.

Ozone Alert for the State of Texas
www.tceq.state.tx.us
Daily ozone alerts can be sent to the user electronically.
(The reader may wish to obtain state or local ozone alert Web site addresses.)

STARBRIGHT Foundation
www.starbright.org
Provides a free educational asthma game for children.

The United States Environmental Protection Agency
www.epa.gov/iaq/schools/
Offers a free indoor air quality tool kit for schools.

GLOSSARY

allergic rhinitis: A hypersensitivity syndrome in which exposure to environmental allergens results in sneezing, nasal pruritis, nasal mucosal edema, rhinorrhea and obstruction.

allergic sensitization: A heightened or exaggerated immune response that develops after more than one exposure to a specific allergen. The response is pathological.

allergen: An antigen that causes an allergic reaction by interacting with antibodies or lymphocytes in patients previously sensitized to that specific antigen.

anticholinergic drug: A drug that impedes the action of fibers of the parasympathetic nerves; used in the treatment of asthma to block the action of acetylcholine at parasympathetic sites in bronchial smooth muscle, causing bronchodilation.

atopy: 1. Derived from the Greek word meaning "strange," the term was introduced into the medical literature in 1923 to describe allergic diseases, such as asthma, atopic dermatitis (eczema), and allergic rhinitis, that have a familial tendency and implied genetic predisposition. Diseases that show no familial tendency are referred to as nonatopic. **2.** A disease with the tendency to produce immunoglobulin (Ig) E.

beta$_2$-agonist: A class of adrenergic agonist agents that act at beta$_2$ sites in the airway to produce bronchodilation. This term is applied to nerve fibers that release epinephrine when stimulated and includes almost all sympathetic fibers.

cytokines: Protein hormones derived from several types of immune cells that are such as lymphocytes, produced when antigens activate immune cells. There are several classes of cytokines, such as the interleukins. Their actions are complex and include nonpathological functions, such as mediation of natural immunity, and pathological functions such as regulation of the immune-mediated inflammatory response in asthma.

eosinophils: Peripheral blood leukocytes comprising 2% to 5% of total leukocytes in healthy individuals. Numbers are increased in airway tissues in individuals with asthma. They are attracted to sites of inflammation by chemotactic factors released by mast cells. Upon degranulation, eosinophils release toxins that destroy airway epithelium and recruit other inflammatory mediators.

epidemiology: The medical science concerned with defining and explaining relationships between host, environment, and agent in causing disease. Epidemiology has contributed to understanding patterns of prevalence of asthma.

hygiene hypothesis: A theory developed to explain differences in rates of asthma among urban and rural dwellers that suggests modern lifestyle, with its emphasis of hygiene and overuse of antibiotics, is thought to lead to an imbalance in the immune system favoring increased numbers of Th2 (inflammatory) cells over Th1 (protective) cells.

hypocapnia: Lack of carbon dioxide in the blood.

INDEX

recommended sources of, 187
Rochester Regional Community Asthma Network,
     181, 183*fig*, 187
See also clients

Y
Yellow zone, 37
yoga, 213, 216-217

Z
Zone concept, 37

PRETEST KEY

Asthma: Nursing Care Across the Lifespan

1.	a	Chapter 1
2.	c	Chapter 2
3.	a	Chapter 3
4.	d	Chapter 4
5.	a	Chapter 5
6.	b	Chapter 5
7.	b	Chapter 6
8.	c	Chapter 6
9.	d	Chapter 7
10.	b	Chapter 7
11.	d	Chapter 8
12.	c	Chapter 9
13.	d	Chapter 9
14.	b	Chapter 10
15.	d	Chapter 11
16.	a	Chapter 12
17.	b	Chapter 13
18.	d	Chapter 14
19.	d	Chapter 15
20.	d	Chapter 16

Notes

Notes

Notes

Notes

Notes

Western Schools® offers over 60 topics to suit all your interests – and requirements!

Clinical Conditions/Nursing Practice

A Nurse's Guide to Weight Control
for Healthy Living ....25 hrs
Airway Management with a Tracheal Tube ....1 hr
Asthma: Nursing Care Across the Lifespan ....28 hrs
Auscultation Skills: Breath and Heart Sounds ......12 hrs
Basic Nursing of Head, Chest, Abdominal,
Spine and Orthopedic Trauma ....16 hrs
Care at the End of Life....................................3 hrs
Chest Tube Management ....2 hrs
Death, Dying & Bereavement ....30 hrs
Diabetes Nursing Care ....30 hrs
Healing Nutrition ....24 hrs
Hepatitis C: The Silent Killer ....2 hrs
HIV/AIDS..1, 2, 4 or 30 hrs
Holistic & Complementary Therapies: Introduction..1 hr
Humor in Healthcare: The Laughter Prescription..20 hrs
Managing Obesity and Eating Disorders ....30 hrs
Nursing Care of the HIV-Infected Patient..............30 hrs
Orthopedic Nursing: Caring for Patients with
Musculoskeletal Disorders ....30 hrs
Pain Management: Principles and Practice............30 hrs
Seizures: A Basic Overview ....1 hr
The Neurological Exam..1 hr
Wound Management and Healing........................30 hrs

Cosmetic Treatments/Surgery

Belt Lipectomy: Lower Body Contouring ....1 hr
Botox Treatments and Dermal Fillers........................1 hr
Cosmetic Breast Surgery ....1 hr
Weight Loss Surgery ....1 hr

Critical Care/ER/OR

Ambulatory Surgical Care ....20 hrs
Case Studies in Critical Care Nursing: A Guide for
Application and Review ....46 hrs
Principles of Basic Trauma Nursing ....30 hrs

Geriatrics

Alzheimer's Disease: A Complete Guide for Nurses ..25 hrs
Alzheimer's: Things a Nurse Needs to Know........12 hrs
Elder Abuse ....4 hrs
Home Health Nursing ....30 hrs
Nursing Care of the Older Adult ....30 hrs
Psychosocial Issues Affecting Older Adults ....16 hrs

**For our free catalog, visit our website
www.westernschools.com
or call today!
1-800-438-8888**

Infectious Diseases/Bioterrorism

Biological Weapons ....5 hrs
Bioterrorism & the Nurse's Response to WMD ......5 hrs
Bioterrorism Readiness: The Nurse's Critical Role .. 2 hrs
Infection Control Training for Healthcare Workers ..4 hrs
Influenza: A Vaccine-Preventable Disease ....1 hr
SARS: An Emerging Public Health Threat ....1 hr
Smallpox..2 hrs
The New Threat of Drug Resistant Microbes ....5 hrs
West Nile Virus ....1 hr

Oncology

Cancer in Women..30 hrs
Cancer Nursing: A Solid Foundation for Practice ..30 hrs
Chemotherapy Essentials: Principles & Practice ..15 hrs

Pediatrics/Maternal-Child/Women's Health

Attention Deficit Hyperactivity Disorders
Throughout the Lifespan...............................30 hrs
Diabetes in Children ....30 hrs
End-of-Life Care for Children and
Their Families ....2 hrs
Manual of School Health....................................30 hrs
Maternal-Newborn Nursing................................30 hrs
Menopause: Nursing Care for Women
Throughout Mid-Life ....25 hrs
Pediatric Nursing: Routine to Emergent Care........30 hrs
Pediatric Pharmacology ....10 hrs
Pediatric Physical Assessment............................10 hrs
Women's Health: Contemporary
Advances and Trends ....30 hrs

Professional Issues/Management/Law

Documentation for Nurses....................................24 hrs
Medical Error Prevention: Patient Safety ....2 hrs
Nursing Practice and the Law ....30 hrs
Nursing and Malpractice Risks:
Understanding the Law ....30 hrs
Ohio Law: Standards of Safe Nursing Practice ....1 hr
Supervisory Skills for Nurses ....30 hrs
Surviving and Thriving in Nursing ....30 hrs
Understanding Managed Care..............................30 hrs

Psychiatric/Mental Health

Antidepressants ....1 hr
Antipsychotics ....1 hr
Anxiolytics and Mood Stabilizers..........................1 hr
Basic Psychopharmacology....................................5 hrs
IPV (Intimate Partner Violence):
A Domestic Violence Concern ....1 or 3 hrs
Psychiatric Principles & Applications for
General Patient Care ....30 hrs
Psychiatric Nursing: Current Trends
in Diagnosis and Treatment ....30 hrs
Substance Abuse ....30 hrs

Visit us online at www.westernschools.com for these great courses – plus all the latest CE topics!
Online testing also available.

REV. 7/24/05